# NLN
# Guide to Success
# on Nursing Examinations

# NLN
# Guide to Success
# on Nursing Examinations

## Leonarda A. Laskevich, RN, MA

Pub. No. 17-2187

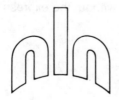

**National League for Nursing • New York**

# Acknowledgements

The first acknowledgement must recognize Harriet Schneider Hess who was responsible for igniting the author's interest in developing tests.

Special thanks and appreciation to Joyce Carusi, NLN Director of Marketing, for her patience and encouragement during the preparation of this book. Without the resources provided by the staff of NLN Test Service, this work could never have been realized. The contributions and content reviews by Gloria Fox, Patricia O'Malley and Elaine Zimbler were of immeasurable value.

Marcia Samuels's careful editing will be especially appreciated by the users of this book. Beverly Rothman, a master word processor, deserves special thanks for performing the tedious task of typing and retyping the first draft and the many revisions of the manuscript.

Appreciation is also extended to the many faculty who spent hours in item writing sessions at NLN and to those who participated in test construction workshops. They contributed to this book by identifying clinical content that was important to include in measuring a nurse's competence in meeting the nursing care needs of patients.

Leonarda A. Laskevich

# About the Author

Leonarda A. Laskevich is a consultant in test development for NLN Test Service, a division of the National League for Nursing which publishes standardized tests for use in nursing education programs and nursing practice. She also conducts workshops on the construction and use of teacher-made tests for faculty in schools of nursing. For many years, Ms. Laskevich was coordinator of the development of the State Board Test Pool Examinations at the National League for Nursing. She is a participating author of a review book for the National Council Licensure Examination for Registered Nurses prepared by the National Council of State Boards of Nursing. Her professional experience includes many years as a faculty member in schools of nursing. She has also held various nursing practice positions, including director of nursing, in acute and long-term care institutions. Ms. Laskevich received her basic nursing education at The Mount Sinai Hospital School of Nursing, New York City, and her B.S. and M.A. degrees from Teachers College, Columbia University, New York.

# Contents

# Contents

# Introduction

This book has been designed as a study guide to assist you in preparing to take the registered nurse licensure examination, NCLEX-RN, as well as other tests used in nursing. The introductory section describes the tests most commonly used—their purpose, scope, and depth—for the benefit of the candidate who is preparing to take a specific examination.

The study guide then provides suggestions about how to prepare for a test and includes a plan for answering the questions that will help you to utilize your study time most efficiently. The study guide also describes the skills that you need to develop as the day approaches to take the scheduled examination.

Hundreds of study questions form the core of the book. The questions are followed by detailed explanations for each patient situation presented. Your responses to the study questions will indicate areas of content that may require further reading; suggested references for each clinical area are provided.

The last section of the study guide is a Comprehensive Test in two sections that can be taken as part of your personal program of study and practice. This test is modeled on the NCLEX-RN test plan.

# Tests in Nursing

Understanding the purpose of a test will help you prepare most effectively. While you are a nursing student, and later as a practicing nurse, you will encounter many different kinds of tests. In schools of nursing, the purpose of testing is generally to assess the knowledge and skills acquired during the educational program. Standardized tests developed by national testing agencies may be used to compare your achievement with the performance of students in schools of nursing throughout the country. Certain standardized tests are used to assess your readiness to take the licensure examination or to determine eligibility for advanced placement in another nursing education program.

To become licensed as a registered nurse, you must successfully complete the National Council Licensure Examination for Registered Nurses, which is often referred to as NCLEX-RN. This examination tests essential nursing knowledge and assesses your ability to provide safe and effective patient care.

During the orientation phase of employment in hospitals and other health care facilities, tests in areas such as pharmacology are frequently administered. In the employment setting, tests are often used for diagnostic purposes, that is to assess competencies in order to plan appropriate inservice education. Tests are also administered to nurses seeking certification in specialty areas of nursing practice. Certification indicates a degree of professional competence that exceeds the requirements for licensure.

## NCLEX-RN

In the United States, nursing is a licensed profession regulated by law. Each state legislature has enacted laws that govern nursing practice in order to protect the public. A Board of Nursing in each state has the responsibility for implementing the law that regulates the practice of nursing in that state and for determining who is eligible for licensure as a registered nurse. A candidate for licensure must meet the specific requirements of the state in which licensure is desired and must successfully complete NCLEX-RN. The licensure examination is developed by the National Council of State Boards of Nursing.

NCLEX-RN tests your ability to apply essential nursing knowledge in patient care situations. The licensure examination is administered twice each year, in February and July, on the same dates throughout the United States. NCLEX-RN is administered in sections, and each part must be completed within a designated period of time. The majority of candidates will have ample time to complete the examination which consists entirely of multiple-choice questions. Each state Board of

Nursing has the responsibility of determining the level of achievement on NCLEX-RN that is required in order to become licensed to practice nursing in that state.

The test plan for NCLEX-RN contains specific criteria that determine the content of the examination. The nursing behaviors identified in the test plan are divided into five broad categories which reflect the steps of the nursing process. These five categories are assessing, analyzing, planning, implementing, and evaluating. The behaviors are the framework within which nursing knowledge is tested in patient care situations.

The patient situations presented include those health problems that the nurse will encounter most frequently. The level of illness or wellness of the patient in the situation will vary and will determine the extent to which the patient can be involved in decisions relating to his or her own care. When a patient is unable to make decisions, the locus of decision-making will be in the nurse. When a patient is in the recuperative and convalescing stages of illness, the patient will usually be involved in decisions about care. In this situation, the locus of decision-making will be shared by the nurse and the patient. When a patient will be managing his own care, the locus of decision-making will be solely in the patient.

Without referring to a specific clinical area, the patient situations will include the nursing care of adults who have common health problems, the nursing care of patients with psychiatric problems, the nursing care of women throughout pregnancy, the nursing care of children, including normal growth and development as well as illnesses common in childhood. The patient situations will include questions that test knowledge of pathophysiology, nursing measures, treatment modalities, and psychosocial aspects of care. The examination includes items at different cognitive levels, with particular emphasis on application and analysis.

The requirements that must be met to practice nursing in a specific state may be obtained by writing to the Board of Nursing in that state.

You may refer to the Registry on pages 231-234 for a listing of the addresses of Boards of Nursing.

## Pre-Licensure Tests

A pre-licensure practice test is frequently administered to nursing students near the end of the educational program. The test includes a sampling of content from the various clinical areas and helps assess your readiness to take NCLEX-RN. Patients with common health problems are described, followed by questions that require the application of nursing knowledge using the nursing process.

As part of your performance report for NLN pre-licensure tests, a total test score is provided which is predictive of your performance on NCLEX-RN. It is important that you understand the information presented on your performance report. Areas of strength and weakness are identified to help you in planning your review for the licensure examination. If you have any questions about the report, be sure to seek the assistance of a faculty member well in advance of the NCLEX examination date.

## CGFNS Qualifying Examination

Graduates of foreign nursing schools who wish to practice nursing in the United States must successfully complete NCLEX-RN in order to become licensed. In addition, a majority of state Boards of Nursing require foreign nurse graduates to pass an examination offered by the Commission on Graduates of Foreign Nursing Schools (CGFNS) prior to taking NCLEX-RN. The CGFNS Qualifying Examination measures nursing knowledge and proficiency in the English language. The examination is given twice each year in many countries around the world and at testing centers in the United States as well. The nursing section of the CGFNS Qualifying Examination is developed according to criteria that are similar to those in the test plan for NCLEX-RN. Graduates of foreign nursing schools should clearly understand that the content of the CGFNS examination reflects the variety of health care situations likely to be encountered by the registered nurse in the United States at the entry level of practice.

Information about the CGFNS Qualifying Examination may be obtained from the Commission on Graduates of Foreign Nursing Schools. You will find the Commission's address in the Registry on page 231.

## NLN Achievement Tests

Many schools of nursing administer NLN achievement tests to measure the attainment of nationally accepted objectives in specific content areas. These standardized tests are developed by faculty representing nursing education programs across the country. NLN achievement tests are usually administered at the completion of a specific course or course sequence. Test results indicate how student achievement compares to that of students in similar types of programs nationwide.

An achievement test designed to measure knowledge in a clinical content area will include descriptions of patients with specific health problems. Each patient care situation is then followed by multiple-choice questions written in the framework of the nursing process. Test questions may relate to pathophysiology, nursing measures, diagnostic tests, treatment modalities, and psychosocial aspects of care.

## Classroom Tests

The curriculum in a school of nursing is designed to ensure that the graduate of the program will be able to function at the entry level of nursing practice by administering safe and effective nursing care. Each course in the program is an essential part of the curriculum

that the faculty considers important in meeting program goals. The objectives of each course will, therefore, reflect a portion of overall program objectives. You will frequently be required to demonstrate how well you have mastered the objectives of a course by responding to questions on a teacher-made test. In planning your review, you should pay particular attention to those areas of course content which your instructor has emphasized.

Types of questions used in a teacher-made test will vary. Test questions may be true-false, completion, matching, essay, multiple-choice, or a combination of some or all of these types. However, most standardized tests that are administered to large numbers of students nationally include only multiple-choice questions. The multiple-choice test is appropriate for assessing level of knowledge, requires a minimum of test-taking skills, and can be easily scored by electronic equipment.

## Challenge Tests

Challenge tests are required by many educational programs in nursing when you are seeking advanced placement. Course credits may be awarded for successful performance on a challenge test. These tests may be prepared by a national testing agency or by the school which requires you to take a challenge examination. The content of the test reflects the objectives of the course for which credit is sought. The school has the responsibility for determining the level of achievement required to obtain advanced placement or credit.

Information about challenge tests is available from the school that offers advanced standing in the nursing program. It is important to obtain as much information as possible about the depth and scope of the content that is included in these examinations. Many standardized placement tests are comprised of multiple-choice questions, but challenge tests developed by the school may include other types of test questions as well.

# Preparing for a Test

Every student enrolled in an educational program is required to demonstrate that learning has taken place. Frequently learning is evaluated and, in some cases, course grades may be determined through use of paper-and-pencil tests. For many persons, years of experience in school does not lessen the anxiety associated with taking a written examination. The overwhelming fear and sense of inadequacy that are often experienced are probably unrealistic but nevertheless a reality. Consider, though, that enrollment in an educational program requires that you attend class and complete specific assignments during which learning has undoubtedly occurred. Successful completion of required courses and graduation from a basic program in nursing are evidence of your achievement. You should have confidence in what you have learned and in your ability to be successful when preparing to take a nationally standardized test in nursing.

Enrollment in a course of study places responsibility on the learner as well as on the teacher. The learner who has a good understanding of the course objectives, attends classes regularly, and pays attention in class will have an important advantage. Success requires that you schedule periods of time for study and review. If your approach to studying had been disorganized, you will experience more intense stress before an examination.

Anxiety can be both a good and a bad influence. A moderate amount of anxiety can increase awareness and improve performance, but when anxiety becomes unmanageable, it cripples efforts to achieve. Extreme anxiety can produce feelings of pressure and apprehension resulting in an inability to concentrate. An assessment of your own feelings will give you a good measure of your level of anxiety. Learning how to control disabling levels of anxiety is critical to success.

Your preparation for an examination should begin as early as possible and should be based on an honest evaluation of your strengths and weaknesses. To plan what should be studied or reviewed, it is important to have a clear understanding of the scope and depth of the knowledge to be tested. The purpose of tests in nursing is to evaluate the extent to which you have the knowledge deemed necessary to provide patients with common health problems the nursing care they require. For each patient problem that the nurse may encounter, the answers to the following questions will serve as a guide for the scope of content that may be included in tests.

1. Are particular characteristics generally present in the person who has a specific health problem?
2. What are the usual symptoms or behaviors that bring the person into the health care system?
3. What information should be obtained at the time of the initial assessment of the person?
4. Does the person require immediate nursing measures?
5. What test will be performed to establish a diagnosis?
6. What is required to prepare the person for diagnostic tests?
7. How is the nurse involved in the care of the person who is having diagnostic tests?
8. What results should be expected for a person with a specific health problem?
9. What are the pathophysiological or psychological alterations that cause the person's problem?
10. What are the nursing diagnoses for a person with a specific health problem?
11. What are the goals of care for this person?
12. How will the goals of care for this person be met?
13. How does the nurse determine if the goals of care are met?
14. Given a medical plan of treatment, what should the nurse know about the plan to meet the nursing needs of the person?

15. What are the possible complications that the person may develop?

16. What comfort measures will the person require through the course of the illness?

17. Does the person require special measures to meet basic needs?

18. What psychosocial needs may the person have?

19. What information does the person need to understand the diagnosis and plan of care?

20. How is the teaching plan developed for the person?

21. How is the effectiveness of a teaching plan evaluated?

22. How is the person's compliance with the prescribed treatment plan determined?

23. What discharge planning is required for that person?

24. What other information about this person is it important for the nurse to know?

Review, not study, may produce better test results. If the material that may be included in the test was well understood at the time it was presented, intensive study of the material will not be required. Review of essential information will help you to gain more rapid recall of the knowledge needed to respond to test questions.

A realistic study schedule must be planned. Not everyone can or needs to set aside the same amount of time. Studying materials thoroughly for short periods over a longer span of time may well produce better results than trying to cram a lot of material into a short period. It is usually better to study at a regular time for no more than one or two hours consecutively. If additional time is required, plan to use odd hours that become available for study. Study time should be spent in learning content that is not well understood. While keeping the outline of questions in mind, read references thoroughly. Making notes and reciting answers to the questions aloud will also help you to remember the information.

The place you select for study and review is important. A quiet place will help you to concentrate and to avoid distractions. Plan to keep in one place your reference books, a dictionary, paper and pencil, and any other materials needed so they will be readily available when your study time begins.

The advisability of studying with one or more other persons will vary with the individual. People have different learning needs, and studying with others may not be most productive for you.

Experience in taking standardized tests may affect test results to some degree. If you have not taken standardized tests before, lack of familiarity may be a real source of anxiety. Review the types of questions included in a test until you are comfortable with them. Most nationally standardized tests in nursing use a multiple-choice format with four options from which to select the answer.

The developers of nursing tests make a sincere effort to avoid questions that require a high degree of skill in test-taking. The questions are clearly stated, and efforts are made to avoid ambiguities in meanings of words or phrases. Each question will have only one answer that is clearly correct. This enables the test-taker to focus on the choices given and, with deductive reasoning, to eliminate incorrect choices and select the correct response.

# Taking a Test

When you are required to take an examination, it is your responsibility to review the procedures for filing the necessary application and paying the appropriate fees. As the date of the examination approaches, check the location of the testing center and determine how you will get there. If overnight accommodations are necessary, they should be arranged well in advance of the test date. It is important to keep all necessary papers—such as your admission ticket—in a safe location to avoid last-minute searching.

Several days before the examination, make a determined effort to get plenty of rest and to be in good physical condition. It is especially important that the day before the test be spent in activities that are pleasant; avoid any stressful situations. Food intake should be simple and wholesome. The evening before the examination should be relaxed; make an effort to get to bed and to sleep early. The examination may be lengthy and require concentration for two hours or more. It is most important to prepare yourself by getting a good night's sleep.

On the day of the examination, allow plenty of time to eat a nourishing breakfast and arrive at the examination site early. Travel delays are not uncommon; plan for them. Arriving at the examination site at the last minute causes unnecessary anxiety, and there is always the possibility that you will arrive too late and be denied admission.

After arriving at the examination site, avoid becoming distracted, especially by the behavior of other examinees who may be experiencing extreme anxiety. If time allows, promote relaxation with measures such as deep-breathing techniques. Maintain confidence in yourself, but recognize that a moderate amount of anxiety can increase your alertness. A good mental attitude is extremely important. On entering the examination room, if you are permitted to select your seat, plan to be close to the front and center of the room. This will better enable you to see and hear the examiner. The directions given at the beginning of the session will often pertain to completing forms that include name, identifying information, and other pertinent data. Listen to the directions and follow them carefully.

Once the test has been distributed, the examiner will usually read aloud the directions for the examination. Read the directions carefully with the examiner and be sure to follow them exactly. Failing to listen attentively or to read directions carefully may create unnecessary difficulties.

Most standardized tests are timed. It is important to pace yourself accordingly. When taking a multiple-choice test, you will usually be allowed an average of one minute to answer each question. Some questions will take only a few seconds to read and answer, while others will take more time. Being prepared with a wristwatch will help you to pace yourself.

Tests that measure knowledge of clinical nursing will usually present a patient/client situation followed by questions about the situation described. Read the description of the patient situation carefully in order to have a good image of the patient. After reading each question, rephrase the question in your own mind to clarify what is being asked. Then read all the choices before selecting your answer. Answer the questions in order. Do not spend too much time on any one question. Make a note of the number of any question for which you are unsure of the answer and proceed with the test.

When the answers are to be recorded on a separate answer sheet, be sure that the number of the question you are answering corresponds to the number on the answer sheet. Caution should be exercised about changing your answer to a multiple-choice question without a good reason. Your first choice of an answer is more likely to be correct than subsequent guesses. When you change answers, it is very important to erase carefully. Most tests will be scored using an electronic scanner that cannot determine the answer intended when erasures are made poorly.

As you proceed with the test, concentrate on the questions. Ignore activity around you, especially when the time allowed for the test is almost over. Other examinees may be leaving the room ahead of you, but finishing the test early does not necessarily mean that the questions have been answered correctly.

When all of the questions to which you selected answers have been completed, go back to the questions that gave you trouble. To guess or not to guess the answer to questions about which you are uncertain depends on knowing beforehand whether the test is to be scored using a formula to correct scores for random guessing. Some standardized tests may be scored by subtracting a fraction for each wrong answer. In this event, greater caution should be taken when guessing the answer. However, reasonable guessing may improve your score. If you do not know the answer to a four-option multiple choice question, reread the question and then determine if one or more choices are wrong. Knowing that certain choices are wrong increases the probability of guessing the correct answer. Guessing among four choices offers only a 25% chance of guessing correctly, but guessing between two choices increases the probability of guessing correctly to 50%.

Before turning in your test materials, it is important to check that all information requested has been completely filled in. Also, check that all stray marks have been erased.

When more than one test is to be taken on the same day, use the period between tests to refresh yourself and prepare for the next examination. It is most important to relax by getting some exercise, to have some light nourishment, and to be sure to use the restroom facilities. Worrying about the results of the first test will increase your anxiety and may interfere with your performance on the second test. When it is time for the second test, proceed with renewed concentration and with confidence in your ability to be successful.

# How to Use This Study Guide

The study questions in this book are divided into sections: **Nursing Care of Adults, Nursing Care During Childbearing, Nursing Care of Children,** and **Psychiatric Nursing.** Select first the clinical area in which you feel the least comfortable. Plan time to answer the study questions, allowing one minute for each question. Then check your answers with the answer key provided, noting the questions that you answered incorrectly. The study questions are followed by explanations for the patient situations presented. Read the explanations carefully, especially those that pertain to patient situations for which you had incorrect answers. Then select a reference to read from

the list of recommended texts at the end of the section. In addition to the references noted, other reference books that you have used in school may be helpful. While reading, outline answers to the questions that have been presented for each patient situation.

This same approach should be used for all the study questions in the other clinical areas. Following this procedure will provide a systematic review of the care of patients with common health problems. You will also gain experience in responding to questions written within the framework of the nursing process.

Once your review of the study questions has been completed, plan to set aside a period of time to complete the Comprehensive Test. After completing the test, check your answers using the key provided.

# NURSING CARE
# OF ADULTS

Directions: Read each study question carefully. Select one answer from the four choices presented that you think answers the question correctly. There is only one correct answer to each question. Use the answer key to find out whether the answer you selected is the correct one. Read carefully the explanations for the patient situations presented in the study questions, paying particular attention to the explanations for any questions you missed.

---

Mr. Charles Abeles, 68 years old, is admitted to the hospital with bacterial pneumonia. He has a history of emphysema.

---

1. Soon after admission, Mr. Abeles begins to have a shaking chill. The nurse should take which of these actions first?

   A. Cover him with a blanket.

   B. Inform the physician about his condition.

   C. Take his temperature.

   D. Offer him a drink of hot fluids.

2. To assist Mr. Abeles in expectorating his respiratory secretions, which of these measures would it be most important to include in his care plan?

   A. Turning Mr. Abeles from side to side every two hours.

   B. Encouraging Mr. Abeles to maintain a high fluid intake.

   C. Monitoring Mr. Abeles's respirations every four hours.

   D. Having Mr. Abeles deep-breathe and cough when his respirations sound moist.

3. Orders for Mr. Abeles include the administration of oxygen by nasal cannula p.r.n. When he requires oxygen, the flow rate should be set at how many liters per minute?

   A. 2

   B. 4

   C. 6

   D. 8

4. Since Mr. Abeles has a history of emphysema, which of these pathophysiologic changes would be consistent with his diagnosis?

   A. Respiratory alkalosis.

   B. Pulmonary vasodilatation.

   C. Increased arterial partial pressure of carbon dioxide.

   D. Increased arterial partial pressure of oxygen.

5. Respiratory therapy is prescribed for Mr. Abeles. The primary purpose of these treatments for him is to

   A. reverse the pathology in his respiratory tract.

   B. promote the expansion of his chest muscles.

   C. stimulate the production of his respiratory secretions.

   D. increase the volume of gas exchange in his alveoli.

---

Mr. Abeles is to have a high-protein, high-calorie diet.

---

6. To encourage Mr. Abeles to increase his food intake, which of these measures should be included in his care plan?

   A. Prompting him to take fluids before eating solid foods.

   B. Allowing him to select the foods he will eat.

   C. Giving him oral care before offering him food.

   D. Assessing his knowledge of good nutrition before explaining the diet prescription.

7. Mr. Abeles is offered snacks that are high in protein. Which of these foods would provide him with the most protein?

   A. Whole-wheat bread with jelly.

   B. Orange juice.

   C. Eggnog.

   D. Cream cheese and crackers.

8. Mr. Abeles asks what he can do to prevent recurring respiratory infections. The nurse should advise him that it would be most important to include which of these measures in his care?

   A. Maintaining a daily exercise program.

   B. Having regular medical examinations.

   C. Remaining indoors when outside temperatures are extremely high or low.

   D. Avoiding contact with persons who are sneezing or coughing.

----------------------------------------
Mr. Abeles is discharged from the hospital, and he attends the clinic.
----------------------------------------

9. Mr. Abeles's arterial blood gases are being analyzed periodically. With advancing emphysema, which of these changes occur?

   A. Decreased $pCO_2$ and increased $pO_2$.

   B. Increased $pCO_2$ and increased $pO_2$.

   C. Decreased $pCO_2$ and decreased $pO_2$.

   D. Increased $pCO_2$ and decreased $pO_2$.

10. Mr. Abeles is assessed for respiratory acidosis. Signs of respiratory acidosis include

    A. restlessness and drowsiness.

    B. sternal retraction and flaring of the nostrils.

    C. pallor and stertorous breathing.

    D. diaphoresis and Kussmaul breathing.

----------------------------------------
A year later, an emphysematous bulla on Mr. Abeles's lung ruptures, and he is admitted to the hospital. A chest tube is inserted and connected to waterseal drainage.
----------------------------------------

11. The purpose of the waterseal drainage for Mr. Abeles is to

    A. raise intrapulmonic pressure.

    B. re-establish subatmospheric intrapleural pressure.

    C. reduce intrapulmonic pressure.

    D. equalize intrapulmonic and intrapleural pressures.

12. While Mr. Abeles has waterseal drainage, the nurse should observe him for signs of tension pneumothorax. Which of these findings are indicative of this complication?

    A. Tracheal shift and unilateral chest movement.

    B. Sternal retraction and moist respirations.

    C. Persistent coughing with expectoration of frothy mucus.

    D. Nasal flaring and flail chest.

----------------------------------------
Mrs. Theresa Kay, 32 years old, is admitted to the hospital because of chronic glomerulo-nephritis. She is weak and lethargic.
----------------------------------------

13. In planning Mrs. Kay's care initially, it is essential to include which of these measures?

    A. Performing active range-of-motion exercises.

    B. Testing a sample of each voiding for the presence of acetone.

    C. Scheduling uninterrupted rest periods.

    D. Restricting daily fluid intake to 2,000 ml.

14. A nurse is to obtain from Mrs. Kay a clean-catch urine specimen. It is essential that the nurse include which of these steps in the procedure for obtaining the specimen?

   A. Obtain the specimen after giving Mrs. Kay a glass of water to drink.

   B. Collect the urine after Mrs. Kay has started the urinary stream.

   C. Place a sponge in the vaginal orifice to avoid contamination of the urine specimen.

   D. Cleanse the perineum with soap and water before collecting all urine voided.

15. The results of which of these laboratory tests will indicate earliest whether Mrs. Kay has renal damage?

   A. Urine specific gravity.

   B. Erythrocyte sedimentation rate.

   C. Serum alkaline phosphatase.

   D. Serum creatinine.

----------------------------------------
Hemodialysis treatments are ordered for Mrs. Kay.
----------------------------------------

16. A purpose of the hemodialysis treatments for Mrs. Kay is to

   A. correct her electrolyte imbalance.

   B. reduce the number of red blood cells in her urine.

   C. increase the filtration rate of fluids in her glomeruli.

   D. reverse the destructive changes in her kidneys.

17. Mrs. Kay's treatment includes receiving sodium heparin. The expected therapeutic effect of heparin for Mrs. Kay is to

   A. dissolve blood clots.

   B. facilitate the breakdown of fibrinogen.

   C. promote the adhesiveness of blood platelets.

   D. interfere with the conversion of prothrombin to thrombin.

18. One day, while Mrs. Kay is having dialysis, she offers many suggestions and reminders to the nurse. Which of these interpretations of Mrs. Kay's behavior would serve as the best basis for an approach by the nurse?

   A. She wants to demonstrate her knowledge about her therapy.

   B. She finds something in the situation that is threatening to her.

   C. She is expressing criticism of the staff.

   D. She is displaying an attitude that is expected of patients in her situation.

19. Mrs. Kay's family tells the nurse that Mrs. Kay seems to become somewhat confused and irritable just before each dialysis treatment. In replying, which information should the nurse convey to Mrs. Kay's family?

   A. Mrs. Kay's symptoms are probably a result of failure to follow dietary restrictions.

   B. Mrs. Kay's symptoms reveal extreme anxiety about having to have the treatment.

   C. Mrs. Kay's symptoms develop when the end products of metabolism accumulate in her blood.

   D. Mrs. Kay's symptoms indicate that she has not adjusted to the treatments.

Mr. Henry Jordan, 46 years old, walks into the emergency room and tells the nurse that he is having severe chest pains. He has a history of a myocardial infarction.

A diagnosis of myocardial infarction is confirmed, and Mr. Jordan is admitted to the coronary care unit. He has an intravenous infusion containing levarterenol (Levophed) bitartrate.

20. After placing Mr. Jordan in a semireclining position, the nurse should take which of these actions next?

A. Determine what he was doing when he developed pain.

B. Start an intravenous infusion.

C. Obtain his vital signs.

D. Take a nursing history.

21. If Mr. Jordan has experienced a myocardial infarction, he will probably give which of these descriptions of his pain?

A. A burning substernal pain after eating a meal high in fats.

B. A stabbing pain in the left chest accompanied by tingling in the fingers.

C. A retrosternal pain radiating to the inner aspects of the arms that is more intense on inspiration and expiration.

D. A sudden onset of substernal pain that is unrelieved by rest.

22. Mr. Jordan is given morphine sulfate intravenously. The desired primary effect of this narcotic for Mr. Jordan is to

A. control his blood pressure.

B. reduce his $O_2$ consumption.

C. stimulate contraction of his cardiac muscles.

D. increase his cardiac output.

23. When Mr. Jordan is brought to the coronary care unit, he appears to be very anxious. The most probable cause of his anxiety is

A. fear of impending death.

B. recollection of his previous heart attack.

C. being hospitalized for a prolonged period.

D. concern over becoming dependent on others.

24. To reduce Mr. Jordan's anxiety, it will be most important that the nurse carry out which of these measures?

A. Explaining to Mr. Jordan that recent life experiences are unrelated to his present condition.

B. Conveying to Mr. Jordan that he is being competently cared for.

C. Informing Mr. Jordan that he will be able to resume full activity in a few weeks.

D. Helping Mr. Jordan to understand that his recovery will depend on his cooperation.

25. Since Mr. Jordan is receiving Levophed, it would be essential to include which of these measures in his care?

A. Measuring each of his voidings.

B. Taking his temperature and counting his respirations at 2-hour intervals.

C. Observing his lower extremities for the development of dependent edema.

D. Monitoring his pulse rate and blood pressure.

26. Mr. Jordan is in cardiogenic shock. His status is caused by which of these pathophysiological alterations?

A. Increased capillary permeability and increased microcirculation.

B. Elevated serum enzymes and depleted blood volume.

C. Decreased function of the left ventricle and tissue hypoxia.

D. Alteration in the extracellular and intracellular ratios of fluid.

27. Mrs. Jordan enters the coronary care unit. She says, "Where is Henry? Is my husband dying?" The nurse should take which of these actions first?

A. Inform Mrs. Jordan about her husband's condition.

B. Take Mrs. Jordan to a quiet area.

C. Permit Mrs. Jordan to go to her husband's bedside.

D. Ask Mrs. Jordan if someone came to the hospital with her.

28. Three hours after Mr. Jordan was admitted, he tells the nurse that his chest pain has recurred. Upon admission, he was given morphine sulfate 15 mg. (gr. 1/4). The medication may be repeated q. 3 to 4h. p.r.n. The nurse should take which of these actions first?

A. Give Mr. Jordan the prescribed narcotic.

B. Place Mr. Jordan in a position of comfort.

C. Ask Mr. Jordan to describe in detail the intensity of the pain.

D. Reassure Mr. Jordan that some pain is to be expected with his condition.

29. On admission, Mr. Jordan's temperature was normal. The next day his temperature rises to 100.4°F. (38°C.). This development is most likely indicative of

A. a low-grade infection.

B. the presence of emboli.

C. the development of atelectasis.

D. an expected reaction of the body to an infarction.

30. On his third hospital day, Mr. Jordan is feeling much better and asks the nurse why his activity is still restricted. When responding, the nurse should include which of these explanations about controlling activity in patients who have had a myocardial infarction?

A. Additional activity at this time is likely to result in respiratory embarrassment.

B. The injured area in the heart is incapable of responding safely at this time to an increase in bodily activity.

C. Complete inactivity is indicated because of the great physical and emotional stress on the heart.

D. Minimal activity promotes the effect of the medication used to control the force of contractions of heart muscle.

---------------------------------------------------
Mr. Jordan's condition improves, and he is transferred to the medical unit. He is tolerating a regular, low-sodium diet.
---------------------------------------------------

31. One evening after a light supper, Mr. Jordan complains of epigastric pain. When assessing Mr. Jordan's complaint, it is most important to consider that he may have which of these problems?

A. An extension of his infarction.

B. Elevated cholesterol levels that are causing gallbladder distress.

C. An increase in gastric motility caused by excitement.

D. Indigestion at the end of the day, which occurs in patients with heart disease.

32. Mr. Jordan likes all of the following beverages. Which one is <u>highest</u> in sodium content?

A. Whole milk.

B. Lemonade.

C. Apple juice.

D. Clear tea.

---

Mrs. Edith Hanson, 56 years old, is admitted to the hospital with cancer of the uterus. She has radium implanted in her uterus. She has an indwelling urinary catheter attached to gravity drainage. Her orders include a low-residue diet.

---

33. Because Mrs. Hanson has radium implanted, the nurse should carry out which of these precautions?

A. Putting on an isolation gown before entering Mrs. Hanson's room.

B. Wearing a mask over the nose and mouth when giving care to Mrs. Hanson.

C. Restricting the time spent at Mrs. Hanson's bedside to giving essential care.

D. Using disposable supplies and equipment for Mrs. Hanson.

34. The chief purpose of the indwelling urinary catheter for Mrs. Hanson is to

A. reduce contamination of the perineum by urine.

B. avoid infection in the kidney.

C. prevent displacement of the radium.

D. minimize exposure of the bowel to radiation.

35. Considering that Mrs. Hanson is on a low-residue diet, she would be permitted to have which of these foods?

A. Whole-grain cereals.

B. Grapefruit sections.

C. Lettuce and tomato salad.

D. Broiled fish.

---

The radium is removed from Mrs. Hanson, and she is to be discharged.

---

36. Mrs. Hanson tells the nurse that her daughter and son-in-law and their two small children visit with her every day. She asks the nurse whether any precautions should be observed when she goes home because of her radiation therapy.

The nurse should give her which of these instructions?

A. "You have no restrictions on your activities when you go home."

B. "The same procedure used here while the radium was in your uterus should be carried out for two days when you are at home."

C. "During your first week at home, it will be advisable for you to limit your contact with your family."

D. "It will be advisable for you to avoid any contact with your grandchildren when you go home."

---
Mrs. Hanson is discharged. Three months later, she has an abdominal hysterectomy and a bilateral salpingo-oophorectomy. Her orders include ambulating on the first postoperative day.
---

37. Postoperative hemorrhage, if it should occur in Mrs. Hanson, would be indicated by which of these alterations in her condition?

    A. A decrease in blood pressure, an increase in pulse rate, and restlessness.

    B. A decrease in blood pressure and pulse rate, and an increase in alertness.

    C. An increase in blood pressure and pulse rate, and lethargy.

    D. An increase in blood pressure, a decrease in pulse rate, and disorientation.


38. To gain Mrs. Hanson's cooperation in carrying out deep-breathing and coughing exercises, the nurse should take which of these measures?

    A. Giving Mrs. Hanson an analgesic as soon as the procedure is completed.

    B. Supporting Mrs. Hanson's abdomen during the procedure.

    C. Reminding Mrs. Hanson of the need for the procedure.

    D. Allowing Mrs. Hanson to select the time that the procedure is to be performed.


39. Mrs. Hanson is told that she should NOT sit for extended periods when she is out of bed. The chief purpose of this instruction is to prevent

    A. constipation.

    B. phlebitis in the lower extremities.

    C. respiratory infection.

    D. stress on the incision.

---
Mr. Edward Gray, 45 years old, has cirrhosis of the liver. He has jaundice and marked ascites when admitted to the hospital. His orders include bed rest.
---

40. Mr. Gray has severe pruritis. To relieve his discomfort, which of these measures should be taken?

    A. Avoiding excessive pressure on his skin when changing his position.

    B. Encouraging him to drink fluids.

    C. Keeping the top bed sheet away from his body by using a cradle.

    D. Applying moisturizing lotion to his body after bathing him with tepid water.


41. Diuretic therapy is ordered for Mr. Gray. The expected effect of the therapy can be assessed most accurately by taking which of these measures daily?

    A. Measuring his abdominal girth.

    B. Weighing him.

    C. Recording his intake and output.

    D. Checking the turgor of his skin.


42. When giving care to Mr. Gray, the nurse detects an odor of alcohol on his breath. The nurse should take which of these actions first?

    A. Tell Mr. Gray of the fatal complications of drinking alcohol.

    B. Ask Mr. Gray where he obtained the alcohol.

    C. Warn Mr. Gray that he is delaying his discharge.

    D. Inform Mr. Gray about the nurse's observation.

Mrs. Peggy Calo, 69 years old, has an eye examination. The physician determines that Mrs. Calo has bilateral cataracts, with the left eye having more advanced changes than the right. She is scheduled for surgery on her left eye in two weeks.

43. Mrs. Calo asks what a cataract is and why the condition is more common in older people. A reply to Mrs. Calo about the cause of cataracts should include which of the following information?

A. Opacity of the pupil develops as a result of a decrease in the elasticity of connective tissue.

B. Loss of transparency of the lens occurs in association with degenerative changes.

C. Density of the vitreous humor develops as a result of the aging process.

D. Cloudiness of the cornea occurs in association with an increased level of glucose in the blood.

44. Mrs. Calo asks the nurse if her surgery could be postponed for a month. The nurse should explain that the delay in surgery would have which of these effects?

A. It might result in irreparable damage to her eyes.

B. It would not alter the outcome.

C. It might necessitate more extensive surgery to remove the cataract.

D. It would result in headaches due to increased intraocular pressure.

Mrs. Calo is admitted to the hospital for extraction of a cataract in her left eye.

45. The nurse observes Mrs. Calo removing a bottle with a prescription label from the drawer in her bedside stand. Mrs. Calo says, "My husband brought me these drops that I've been using for several months, ever since I first saw my eye doctor. I've had the prescription refilled several times."

It would be most important for the nurse to ask Mrs. Calo which of these questions first?

A. "How do you put the drops in your eyes?"

B. "When do you use the drops?"

C. "What is the name of the drops?"

D. "Who is the physician who prescribed the drops?"

Mrs. Calo has the surgery as planned. Her left eye is covered with a dressing and an eye shield. Her orders include propoxyphene hydrochloride (Darvon) every 4 hours p.r.n.

46. In the immediate postoperative period, it would be most important to include which of these measures in Mrs. Calo's care?

A. Measuring Mrs. Calo's urinary output.

B. Positioning Mrs. Calo on her affected side.

C. Having Mrs. Calo cough deeply.

D. Determining if Mrs. Calo has nausea.

47. Mrs. Calo complains of sharp pain in her left eye. The nurse should take which of these actions first?

A. Notify the physician.

B. Administer the prescribed analgesic to Mrs. Calo.

C. Examine Mrs. Calo's affected eye.

D. Tell Mrs. Calo to close the lids of both eyes.

---
Mrs. Calo is to be discharged and is to return to the clinic for follow-up care.
---

48. Mrs. Calo's discharge instructions should include which of these precautions?

    A. "Avoid activities involving lifting."

    B. "Refrain from watching television."

    C. "Turn your eyes rather than your head when focusing on objects."

    D. "Rest frequently."

49. The physician prescribes temporary glasses for Mrs. Calo. Which of these effects should be expected in the sight of her operated eye when she obtains the glasses?

    A. All perceived objects will appear to have halos.

    B. Central vision will be better than peripheral vision.

    C. Vision will be sharpest in dimly lighted areas.

    D. True color will not be perceived.

---
Mr. Mark Keller, 21 years old, is brought to the emergency room by ambulance. His history reveals that he hit his head on the ground when he was thrown forward in a motorcycle accident. It is suspected that he has a fracture of cervical vertebrae.
---

50. When Mr. Keller arrives in the emergency room, which of these actions should be carried out first?

    A. Remove Mr. Keller's clothing.

    B. Ask Mr. Keller how to contact his next of kin.

    C. Ascertain the extent to which Mr. Keller can move his extremities.

    D. Assess Mr. Keller's respirations.

51. Mr. Keller is observed for early symptoms of increased intracranial pressure. Which of these changes in his vital signs would be indicative of an increase in intracranial pressure?

    A. Increased blood pressure and decreased pulse rate.

    B. Increased blood pressure and increased pulse rate.

    C. Decreased blood pressure and increased pulse rate.

    D. Decreased blood pressure and decreased pulse rate.

---
A diagnosis of a concussion and fractures of the lower cervical and upper thoracic vertebrae is made. Skeletal traction is applied to Mr. Keller. He is admitted to the surgical unit.
---

52. Which of these symptoms, if it were to develop in Mr. Keller, should be reported immediately?

    A. Spasm of left great toe.

    B. Urinary output of 35 ml. per hour.

    C. Slurring of speech.

    D. Increase in body temperature from 98ºF. (36.7ºC.) at 8 a.m. to 100.8ºF. (38.2ºC.) at 4 p.m.

53. After several weeks the skeletal traction is removed, and Mr. Keller is to be allowed out of bed in a chair. Before Mr. Keller gets out of bed for the first time, which of these measures would prevent orthostatic hypotension?

    A. Strengthening his leg muscles with active exercise.

    B. Raising the head of his bed gradually to high-Fowler's position.

    C. Teaching him deep-breathing exercises.

    D. Moving him by the logrolling technique.

Mrs. Nora Butler, 42 years old, has had rheumatic heart disease for many years. She has become increasingly incapacitated and has limited tolerance of physical activity. She is admitted to the hospital for an evaluation for a possible mitral valve replacement.

54. Since Mrs. Butler has mitral stenosis of rheumatic origin, the pathophysiologic alteration has probably caused which of these characteristic changes in the structure of her heart?

   A. The aortic and tricuspid valves have lost elasticity.

   B. The pulmonary and aortic valves have become constricted by bacterial growth.

   C. The flaps of the tricuspid valve have fused.

   D. The bicuspid valve has become calcified.

55. Mrs. Butler has a cardiac catheterization. This procedure is expected to provide which of the following information about Mrs. Butler's cardiac status?

   A. The adequacy of the conduction system of her heart.

   B. The carbon dioxide content of her atria and the oxygen-carbon dioxide ratio in her coronary arteries.

   C. The oxygen concentration and the pressure of the blood within various chambers of her heart.

   D. The adequacy of the blood supply to her heart muscle.

56. Since Mrs. Butler has mitral stenosis, the backflow of blood occurs into which of these structures first?

   A. Right ventricle.

   B. Left atrium.

   C. Coronary vessels.

   D. Aorta.

57. Mrs. Butler expresses intense concern about getting in a draft and catching cold. She comes close to tears if a window or door is opened. Which of these interpretations of Mrs. Butler's behavior is probably most justifiable?

   A. She is testing the staff's acceptance of her prior to surgery.

   B. She is trying to keep the staff close at hand to promote her security.

   C. She is dealing with her anxiety by means of displacement.

   D. She is demonstrating an understanding of the possible complications of cardiac surgery.

Mrs. Butler is scheduled for a surgical replacement of her mitral valve.

58. In preparing Mrs. Butler for postoperative deep-breathing and coughing exercises, the nurse should give her which of these instructions?

   A. "Take several deep breaths, then tighten your abdominal muscles and cough forcefully."

   B. "Lean backward, take a deep breath, and cough forcefully."

   C. "Lie on your right side, take a deep breath, and cough forcefully."

   D. "Exhale forcefully with your mouth open, and then cough several times."

Mrs. Butler has her mitral valve replaced. When she is returned to her unit, her chest tube is attached to a waterseal drainage system that is connected to suction.

59. While chest suction is being used with the waterseal drainage system for Mrs. Butler, her nursing care should include which of these objectives?

   A. To prevent outside air from entering into the system.

   B. To maintain the intermittent flow of drainage.

   C. To increase negative pressure within the drainage system.

   D. To restrict the expansion of her chest wall by using pillow splints.

60. Several days after her surgery, Mrs. Butler says to the nurse, "The doctor told me that my operation was successful. Does that mean that I can finally do all the things I've wanted to do for so long?" The nurse's initial response should be which of these statements?

   A. "You can probably do most of the things that you've wanted to do, but there will be some restrictions."

   B. "Although your operation was successful, no prediction can be made about the type of activities you'll be permitted."

   C. "The ability to be more active seems to mean a great deal to you. I'd like to hear what kinds of activities you have in mind."

   D. "I can't answer that question myself. You'll have to discuss it with your doctor."

Mr. Edward Lawrence, 76 years old, is admitted to the hospital with symptoms of benign prostatic hypertrophy. His orders include an intravenous pyelogram (IVP).

61. Persons who have prostatic hypertrophy usually develop which of these symptoms first?

   A. Sensation of rectal pressure when voiding.

   B. Dark reddish-brown colored urine.

   C. Inability to completely empty the bladder.

   D. Lower abdominal cramps after urination.

62. Following the IVP, it would be most important to include which of these measures in Mr. Lawrence's care?

   A. Monitoring the volume of his voidings.

   B. Taking his temperature every 4 hours.

   C. Encouraging him to cough at regular intervals.

   D. Having him drink fluids frequently.

The results of the diagnostic studies reveal that Mr. Lawrence has benign prostatic hypertrophy. He has a transurethral prostatectomy under spinal anesthesia. When he is returned to the surgical unit, he has an indwelling urethral catheter attached to gravity drainage.

63. Because Mr. Lawrence has had spinal anesthesia, he should be placed in which of these positions initially?

   A. Semi-Fowler's.

   B. High-Fowler's.

   C. Side-lying.

   D. Supine.

---
Mr. Lawrence's condition improves, and his urethral catheter is removed.
---

64. Mr. Lawrence is observed for evidence of urinary retention. Which of these assessments would provide the most reliable data?

   A. The glucose content of his urine.

   B. The amount of urine he voids during each 24-hour period.

   C. The color and odor of his urine.

   D. The time and amount of each of his voidings.


65. Mr. Lawrence is receiving dioctyl sodium sulfosuccinate (Colace). This medication is expected to have which of these effects?

   A. Lubricating his intestinal tract.

   B. Softening his stools.

   C. Increasing his intestinal peristalsis.

   D. Relieving his flatus.


---
Miss Carol Dunn, 17 years old, is brought to the emergency room by her parents after they discovered that Miss Dunn had ingested an unknown number of barbiturate capsules. She is becoming increasingly unresponsive to verbal stimuli.
---

66. Upon Miss Dunn's arrival in the emergency room, which of these actions should the nurse take first?

   A. Obtain a urine specimen from Miss Dunn.

   B. Assess Miss Dunn's respirations.

   C. Prepare to aspirate Miss Dunn's gastric contents.

   D. Take Miss Dunn's blood pressure.


---
Miss Dunn is admitted to the hospital. Her orders include an intravenous infusion and an indwelling urinary catheter that is attached to gravity drainage.
---

67. The primary purpose of Miss Dunn's indwelling urinary catheter is to

   A. prevent urinary incontinence.

   B. assess the adequacy of hydration.

   C. monitor renal function.

   D. determine the rate of barbiturate excretion.


68. Miss Dunn becomes restless and tries to get out of bed over the side rails. The nurse should take which of these actions first?

   A. Calm Miss Dunn by talking quietly to her.

   B. Assess Miss Dunn's orientation.

   C. Call for assistance in protecting Miss Dunn from injury.

   D. Put a body restraint on Miss Dunn.


69. Several hours later, when the nurse calls Miss Dunn by name, Miss Dunn responds for the first time by mumbling incoherently. The nurse's reply should include which of these statements?

   A. "You can help us by explaining what is troubling you."

   B. "You are getting better and your parents will be very happy."

   C. "You are in a hospital and I am your nurse."

   D. "You are ill after taking an overdose of barbiturates."

70. Miss Dunn's condition improves. She says to the nurse, "Why didn't I die? I'll never be able to take those exams." She then begins to sob. Which of these actions by the nurse would be most important at this time?

A. Remain quietly with Miss Dunn.

B. Explore with Miss Dunn her feelings about death.

C. Ask Miss Dunn about her academic record.

D. Explain to Miss Dunn the importance of being hopeful when faced with a stressful situation.

---

Mr. Sam Paulson, 39 years old, has recurring symptoms of a peptic ulcer. He is admitted to the hospital for diagnostic studies and further treatment. His orders include ambulation as desired and a gastroscopy.

---

71. Mr. Paulson has the gastroscopy. Immediately following the procedure, it would be essential to include which of these measures in his care?

A. Keeping him in a supine position to promote drainage of saliva.

B. Giving him nothing by mouth until his gag reflex returns.

C. Offering him warm saline gargles to prevent hoarseness.

D. Maintaining him on bed rest until he has had sufficient rest.

---

The results of the diagnostic studies confirm the presence of a large gastric ulcer. Mr. Paulson has a subtotal gastrectomy. When he is returned to the surgical unit, he has a nasogastric tube connected to low, intermittent suction.

---

72. Immediately after surgery, the nurse should expect Mr. Paulson's nasogastric tube drainage to be which of these colors?

A. Yellow.

B. Green.

C. Dark red.

D. Light brown.

73. Since Mr. Paulson has a nasogastric tube, which of these measures would most likely be included in his immediate postoperative care?

A. Applying a water-soluble lubricant to his nares.

B. Offering him sips of water.

C. Irrigating the nasogastric tube with sterile saline every three hours.

D. Clamping the nasogastric tube for one-half hour every four hours.

---

Mr. Paulson's condition improves. His nasogastric tube and intravenous infusion are removed. He progresses to a bland diet.

---

74. Mr. Paulson is taught about the possible development of a dumping syndrome. Which of these symptoms is characteristic of this condition?

A. Vomiting.

B. Abdominal pain.

C. Weakness.

D. Abdominal distention.

Mrs. Eva Martin, 46 years old, is brought to the emergency room with burns of the upper chest, neck, face, and both hands and arms. Most of her burns are third degree. Mrs. Martin sustained her injury when a small gas heater exploded.

75. Mrs. Martin is given morphine sulfate intravenously. The narcotic is administered intravenously rather than subcutaneously primarily to achieve which of these purposes?

A. To provide relief of pain.

B. To hasten absorption of the drug.

C. To maintain the integrity of the remaining skin surface.

D. To control routes of entry for organisms.

76. Since Mrs. Martin has severely burned areas, she may develop oliguria due to which of these physiological alterations?

A. Decreased carbonic anhydrase.

B. Decreased release of aldosterone.

C. Decreased hematocrit.

D. Decreased blood pressure.

Mrs. Martin is admitted to the hospital. Most of her burned areas are to be treated by the exposure method.

77. The primary goal of the exposure method of treatment used for Mrs. Martin is to

A. control pain.

B. reduce odor.

C. prevent contractures.

D. inhibit bacterial growth.

78. Twenty-four hours after admission, the nurse obtains all of the following data on Mrs. Martin. Which finding most clearly indicates that Mrs. Martin is developing kidney failure?

A. Decreasing level of consciousness.

B. Albuminuria.

C. Average urinary output of 15 ml. an hour.

D. Serum potassium, 4 mEq/L.

79. All of the following measures are included in Mrs. Martin's care. Which one should have priority?

A. Changing her position.

B. Maintaining the prescribed infusion rate of fluids for her.

C. Providing her with emotional support.

D. Relieving her pain.

Mr. Ray Graham, 78 years old, has been having episodes of transient cerebral ischemia. He is admitted to the hospital for diagnostic tests.

80. The nurse should assess Mr. Graham for symptoms that are common during an episode of transient cerebral ischemia. These symptoms include

A. confusion, vertigo, and muscular weakness.

B. epistaxis, ringing in the ears, and excessive talkativeness.

C. tinnitus, unsteady gait, and fine tremors.

D. nausea, projectile vomiting, and inappropriate affect.

81. All of these goals would be appropriate for the nursing care plans of all patients. Which one should have priority in Mr. Graham's care?

A. Adequate nutrition.

B. Preservation of skin integrity.

C. Protection against injury.

D. Maintenance of privacy.

---

Mr. Graham has a carotid angiogram.

---

82. The purpose of a carotid angiogram for Mr. Graham is to

A. determine if there is an obstruction of the circulation within the intracranial vessels.

B. estimate the rate of cerebral venous flow.

C. visualize the aorta and coronary blood vessels.

D. identify cardiopulmonary blood flow.

---

Mrs. Sara Warner, 79 years old, falls in her home and sustains a fracture of the head of the femur of her right hip. She is admitted to the hospital and scheduled to have a surgical repair. Skin traction (Buck's extension) is to be applied to her right leg.

---

83. Before the Buck's extension is applied, which of these assessments of Mrs. Warner would be essential?

A. When did Mrs. Warner last eat?

B. What is the condition of the skin of Mrs. Warner's affected leg?

C. What allergies has Mrs. Warner experienced in the past?

D. When did Mrs. Warner last wash her legs and feet?

84. While Mrs. Warner's right leg is in Buck's extension, her care plan should include which of these measures?

A. Placing a sandbag along the calf of her right leg.

B. Keeping the skin of her right heel intact.

C. Maintaining the sole of her right foot against a footboard.

D. Positioning a pillow under her right thigh.

85. Mrs. Warner complains that the traction is causing a pulling sensation in her right leg. The nurse should give Mrs. Warner which of these explanations?

A. "The pull on your leg is necessary to prevent futher injury. I will check that the traction is in good order."

B. "Try bending your knee at least once an hour to ease the pull of the traction on your leg. I will show you how to do it."

C. "I'll take some weight off the traction for a short while. That will give you a little rest."

D. "I'll raise your foot a few inches. That will relieve some of your discomfort from the traction."

86. Mrs. Warner makes repeated requests for the nurse to rearrange her bedside table. Whenever the nurse finishes doing what Mrs. Warner requested and begins to leave the room, Mrs. Warner makes additional requests.

The nurse should make which of these interpretations of Mrs. Warner's behavior?

A. Mrs. Warner is looking for companionship.

B. Mrs. Warner is displaying actions that are common to elderly persons.

C. Mrs. Warner is forgetting what she really wants to request.

D. Mrs. Warner is anxious about what is happening to her.

Mrs. Warner has a surgical replacement of the head of her right femur. When she is brought back to her room, her condition is stable, and she has an intravenous infusion.

---

87. To maintain the integrity of the surgical procedure, Mrs. Warner's care plan should include which of these measures?

    A. Keeping the affected extremity slightly abducted.

    B. Exercising the affected extremity passively.

    C. Placing the foot of the affected extremity on a pillow.

    D. Flexing the affected extremity when changing position from side to side.

88. Three hours after Mrs. Warner is back in her room, she develops moist respirations and she is slightly dyspneic. The nurse should take which of these actions first?

    A. Slow the flow rate of the intravenous infusion.

    B. Prepare to administer oxygen.

    C. Auscultate the chest.

    D. Encourage deep-breathing exercises.

89. To prepare Mrs. Warner for ambulation, her care plan includes teaching her quadriceps-setting exercises. The teaching should include giving her which of these instructions?

    A. "Squeeze your buttocks together while crossing and uncrossing your legs."

    B. "While lying on your back, keep the back of your knee against the bed and try to lift your heel."

    C. "Rotate your ankle while flexing and extending your foot."

    D. "Flex your hip and, keeping your foot flat on the bed, swing your knee back and forth."

---

Mr. Mark Hinton, 32 years old, has diabetes mellitus, which has just been diagnosed. He is being seen in the clinic. His orders include isophane (NPH) insulin and a diet using the exchange list. The nurse develops a teaching plan for Mr. Hinton.

---

90. When beginning to teach Mr. Hinton about his condition, the nurse should take which of these actions first?

    A. Have Mr. Hinton talk to another patient who has diabetes.

    B. Provide Mr. Hinton with literature about diabetes.

    C. Determine what Mr. Hinton knows about diabetes.

    D. Ask Mr. Hinton how many members of his family have diabetes.

91. Mr. Hinton should be taught that which of these activities requires a preventive measure to avoid a hypoglycemic reaction?

    A. Exercising strenuously.

    B. Eating unsweetened grapefruit.

    C. Having breakfast five minutes after injecting insulin.

    D. Failing to test urine for glucose upon arising.

92. Mr. Hinton should recognize which of these symptoms as an early sign of hypoglycemia?

    A. Feeling of tremulousness.

    B. Flushing of the face and neck.

    C. Sudden onset of fatigue.

    D. Thirst.

93. Mr. Hinton would demonstrate understanding of the use of the food exchange list if he selected which of these foods as an appropriate exchange for white rice?

A. Raisins.

B. Carrot.

C. Celery.

D. Bread.

94. Mr. Hinton tells the nurse that he does not like tuna fish. He should be instructed that which of these foods is an appropriate exchange for a serving of tuna fish?

A. An egg.

B. A peanut butter sandwich.

C. One portion of buttered noodles.

D. Two strips of bacon.

95. Since Mr. Hinton is to take NPH insulin, he should be taught that he may have a hypoglycemic reaction at which of these times?

A. Before breakfast.

B. Midmorning.

C. Late afternoon.

D. Early evening.

---

Four months later Mr. Hinton develops a gastrointestinal infection. After three days of vomiting and diarrhea, he is brought to the emergency room. After being examined, he is admitted to the hospital in ketoacidosis. An intravenous infusion of normal saline is started, and he is to receive regular insulin subcutaneously.

---

96. Since Mr. Hinton is in ketoacidosis, the results of his blood tests will show which of these alterations in his acid-base balance?

A. The pH will be elevated.

B. The hydrogen ion concentration will be increased.

C. The bicarbonate level will be higher than normal.

D. The potassium level will be rising.

97. Information about Mr. Hinton's buffering system will be provided by the results of which of these blood studies?

A. Serum glucose.

B. Leukocyte count.

C. Hematocrit.

D. Serum carbon dioxide.

98. Mr. Hinton responds to treatment, and when the results of his blood studies are approaching normal, an intravenous solution containing glucose is prescribed. The glucose solution is expected to achieve which of these results?

A. Control elimination of carbonic acid.

B. Increase absorption of insulin.

C. Prevent hypoglycemia.

D. Provide a source of energy.

Mrs. Helen Nadler, 66 years old, has hypertension. She attends the medical clinic.

99. Mrs. Nadler's hypertension is most probably related to which of these pathophysiological alterations?

A. Dilation of renal arteries.

B. Spasms of venules.

C. Loss of elasticity in arterioles.

D. Depletion of serum calcium.

100. The nurse discusses health maintenance with Mrs. Nadler. It would be most important at this time for the nurse to make which of these assessments?

A. Does Mrs. Nadler have a knowledge of good body mechanics?

B. Does Mrs. Nadler follow a regular physical activity program?

C. Does Mrs. Nadler eat a diet that is well balanced?

D. Does Mrs. Nadler have stressful situations in her life?

101. Mrs. Nadler is given instruction about restricting sodium in her diet. Which of these statements, if made by Mrs. Nadler, would indicate that she needs further instruction?

A. "I can have a slice of white toast with jelly for breakfast."

B. "I will use a salad dressing made with oil and lemon juice."

C. "I'm glad I can add soy sauce when stir-frying vegetables."

D. "I'll start drinking tea that is decaffeinated."

Six months later Mrs. Nadler is brought to the emergency room. She has dyspnea and edema of the lower extremities. Following examination, she is admitted to the hospital with congestive heart failure. Her orders include bed rest, digoxin (Lanoxin), furosemide (Lasix), and blood tests.

102. When Mrs. Nadler is admitted, the nurse should carry out which of these measures first?

A. Obtaining a nursing history from Mrs. Nadler.

B. Starting an intravenous infusion for Mrs. Nadler.

C. Elevating Mrs. Nadler's legs on a pillow.

D. Placing Mrs. Nadler in a semi-Fowler's position.

103. Since Mrs. Nadler has edema of the lower extremities, her care plan should include which of these measures?

A. Applying lotion to her legs.

B. Limiting her intake of fluids.

C. Changing her position every 2 hours.

D. Having her wear elastic stockings.

104. Mrs. Nadler is to receive Lanoxin 0.5 mg. p.o. Lanoxin is available in 0.25 mg. tablets. How many tablets should she be given?

A. 1

B. 2

C. 3

D. 4

105. To assess Mrs. Nadler for possible side effects of Lanoxin, the nurse should ask her which of these questions?

A. "Have your bowel habits changed?"

B. "Do you have any ringing in your ears?"

C. "What is the color of your urine?"

D. "Has your appetite changed?"

106. When the desired therapeutic effects of Lanoxin have been achieved for Mrs. Nadler, the nurse will obtain which of the following data about Mrs. Nadler's condition?

A. Her pulse rate has increased.

B. Her pulse pressure has decreased.

C. Her pulse is stronger.

D. Her apical and radial pulse rates are the same.

107. While Mrs. Nadler is receiving Lasix, she should be served foods that are high in which of these nutrients?

A. Vitamin B.

B. Vitamin C.

C. Potassium.

D. Calcium.

108. The achievement of the desired therapeutic effect of Lasix would be most strongly indicated by which of these changes in Mrs. Nadler's condition?

A. Increased appetite.

B. Weight loss.

C. Decreased ankle edema.

D. Strengthened heart contractions.

109. Mrs. Nadler is assessed for symptoms of hypokalemia, which include

A. arrhythmia.

B. oliguria.

C. restlessness.

D. peripheral neuritis.

---

Mr. Eric Granger, 64 years old, has peripheral vascular disease. He complains of symptoms in his lower extremities. He is admitted to the hospital for an arteriogram and possible surgery.

---

110. When Mr. Granger's nursing history is being taken, which of these questions should he be asked to determine if he has had intermittent claudication?

A. "How far can you walk without discomfort in your legs?"

B. "Can you climb two flights of stairs without becoming short of breath?"

C. "Do you feel more comfortable sitting with your legs elevated than with your feet resting on the floor?"

D. "Are your feet swollen when you take your shoes off at the end of a day?"

111. When performing a physical assessment of Mr. Granger, the nurse should expect to observe symptoms of peripheral vascular disease, which include

A. complaints of dizziness upon rising to a standing position.

B. prominent popliteal varicosities.

C. ankle edema.

D. feet that feel cold to the touch.

112. When preparing Mr. Granger for the arteriogram, it is most important to take which of these measures?

A. Wrapping his legs with elastic bandage.

B. Encouraging him to have a high fluid intake.

C. Obtaining a history of his allergies.

D. Shaving his lower extremities.


113. Mr. Granger's care should be based on which of these nursing diagnoses?

A. Tissue ischemia related to poor oxygen transport.

B. Venous stasis related to atrophy of leg muscles.

C. Potential for thrombus formation related to vascular congestion.

D. Potential for development of leg ulcer related to loss of skin turgor.


114. Which of these goals of care would be most important for Mr. Granger?

A. To increase the circulation to his legs with exercise.

B. To detect signs of injury to his legs with daily inspection.

C. To promote muscle strength in his legs with massage.

D. To monitor vascular resistance in his legs with daily blood pressure determinations.

---

The results of diagnostic tests reveal that Mr. Granger has extreme narrowing of the femoral artery in the midthigh area of his left leg. He has a femoral bypass graft. When he is brought to his room, he has an intravenous infusion running. Mr. Granger's wife is visiting him.

---

115. Mrs. Granger asks the nurse when her husband's intravenous infusion will be discontinued. The nurse should inform her that the intravenous infusion will probably be discontinued at which of these times?

A. When Mr. Granger's left pedal pulse is of good quality.

B. When Mr. Granger's foot begins to feel warm to the touch.

C. When Mr. Granger is able to tolerate fluids by mouth.

D. When Mr. Granger's blood pressure is approximately the same as his preoperative blood pressure.

---

Ms. Marilyn Onley, 22 years old, has pharyngitis that has not responded to treatment. She is seen in the clinic, and results of blood tests indicate that she may have leukemia. She is admitted to the hospital for further diagnostic tests including a bone marrow aspiration.

---

116. The report of Ms. Onley's blood tests includes the following results: hemoglobin, 9.6 gm./dl.; hematocrit, 31%; and leukocyte count, 50,000 per cu. mm. Which of these interpretations of this data would be correct?

A. The hemoglobin and hematocrit are within normal limits, and the white cell count is low.

B. The hemoglobin is low, and the hematocrit and white cell count are within normal limits.

C. The hemoglobin and white cell count are within normal limits, and the hematocrit is high.

D. The hemoglobin, hematocrit, and white cell count are abnormal findings.

117. Ms. Onley is informed when she will have the bone marrow aspiration. She begins to cry and says, "I'm so frightened." In response to Ms. Onley, the nurse should make which of these remarks?

A. "The procedure is brief and painless."

B. "You will receive a local anesthetic for the procedure."

C. "I would like to know what is concerning you about the procedure."

D. "The doctor will explain each step of the procedure as it is done."

118. Before Ms. Onley has the bone marrow aspiration, the nurse should take which of these actions?

A. Ask Ms. Onley to empty her bladder.

B. Determine if Ms. Onley has signed a consent form.

C. Check that Ms. Onley has taken nothing by mouth for 4 hours.

D. Take Ms. Onley's vital signs.

---

The results of diagnostic tests confirm that Ms. Onley has acute myelogenous leukemia. Her treatment is to include methotrexate, mercaptopurine (Purinethol), and vincristine sulfate (Oncovin).

---

119. Ms. Onley's initial plan of care should give priority to which of these goals?

A. To conserve her energy.

B. To provide her with information about her condition.

C. To include her in managing her care.

D. To encourage diversional activities.

---

After Ms. Onley receives the initial chemotherapy treatment, she is discharged from the hospital, and treatment is continued on an outpatient basis.

---

120. Ms. Onley develops stomatitis. The nurse should advise her to use which of these methods of oral hygiene?

A. Rinse her mouth with a mild alkaline solution.

B. Apply gentian violet to ulcerated areas in her mouth.

C. Swab her mouth with a mixture of glycerine and lemon juice.

D. Coat her mouth with mineral oil.

121. Since Ms. Onley is receiving chemotherapy, it is most important that she include which of these measures in her care?

A. Eating foods high in potassium.

B. Using a humidifier when sleeping.

C. Avoiding crowds.

D. Stimulating her scalp with brushing.

122. Because of the immunosuppressive effects of chemotherapy, Ms. Onley should be instructed to report the development of which of these symptoms without delay?

A. Pallor.

B. Lethargy.

C. Diarrhea or constipation.

D. Chills and fever.

Mr. Edward Ross, 67 years old, is admitted to the hospital and has a biopsy of a tumor on the larynx. The results of the biopsy reveal that he has cancer of the larynx. Mr. Ross is informed, and he consents to a laryngectomy.

123. The next day Mr. Ross says to the nurse, "My wife and my brother both died of cancer. They both suffered for such a long time." Which of these responses by the nurse would be most therapeutic at this time?

A. Explain to Mr. Ross that the treatment of cancer has become much more effective in prolonging life.

B. Encourage Mr. Ross to continue to express his thoughts.

C. Ask Mr. Ross for the details of his relatives' illness.

D. Determine from Mr. Ross what concerns him about having cancer.

124. Mr. Ross's preoperative preparation should most certainly include which of these measures?

A. Establishing a method of communication to use postoperatively.

B. Describing the type of equipment that will be used in his postoperative care.

C. Explaining the type of nourishment he will receive postoperatively.

D. Informing him that visitors will be restricted in the early postoperative period.

Mr. Ross has a total laryngectomy. When he is brought to the surgical intensive care unit, he has a laryngectomy tube in place.

125. During the procedure for suctioning through Mr. Ross's laryngectomy tube, suction should be applied at which of these times?

A. When the catheter is being inserted and removed.

B. When the catheter is in the trachea but not when it is being inserted or removed.

C. When the catheter is being removed but not when it is being inserted.

D. When the catheter is being inserted and while it is in the trachea.

Mr. Ernest Jackson, 72 years old, is admitted to the hospital with a cerebrovascular accident. He has paralysis of the left side. He is in a coma and responds to painful stimuli.

126. Mr. Jackson's care plan should include measures to prevent complications. Which of these complications poses an early risk for him?

A. Contractures.

B. Loss of skin integrity.

C. Cystitis.

D. Upper respiratory infection.

127. Which of these measures in Mr. Jackson's care should receive priority?

A. Measuring his urinary output.

B. Changing his position at regular intervals.

C. Performing passive range-of-motion exercises.

D. Providing verbal stimuli.

128. Nasogastric tube feedings are ordered for Mr. Jackson. Feedings should be administered at a slow rate for which of these purposes?

A. To prevent aspiration from regurgitation.

B. To allow normal absorption of nutrients.

C. To prevent diarrhea.

D. To stimulate gastric secretions.

---

Mrs. Fay Inwood, 39 years old, goes to a health maintenance clinic for the first time.

---

129. Among the data that the nurse collects from a physical assessment of Mrs. Inwood are the following:

   Weight, 140 lb. (63.6 kg.)
   Height, 5 ft. 1 in. (154.5 cm.)
   Blood pressure, 140/90

Before Mrs. Inwood leaves the clinic, it would be most important for the nurse to take which of these actions?

A. Take Mrs. Inwood's blood pressure again.

B. Reweigh Mrs. Inwood on another scale.

C. Advise Mrs. Inwood to reduce the carbohydrate content of her diet.

D. Tell Mrs. Inwood to restrict her diet to foods that are low in sodium.

130. All women who attend the clinic are taught breast self-examination. When planning Mrs. Inwood's teaching program, the nurse should use which of these approaches initially?

A. Encourage Mrs. Inwood to ask questions about breast self-examination.

B. Give Mrs. Inwood literature about breast self-examination.

C. Show Mrs. Inwood a teaching film about breast self-examination.

D. Ascertain what Mrs. Inwood knows about breast self-examination.

131. When Mrs. Inwood examines the medial half of her left breast, she should place her left hand at which of these sites?

A. On her abdomen.

B. Beneath her back.

C. Under her head.

D. By her side.

132. Mrs. Inwood leaves the clinic. A few months later, she feels a lump in her breast. She returns to the clinic and tells the nurse about the lump and that she expects her menstrual period in 5 days. The nurse should take which of these actions?

A. Suggest to Mrs. Inwood that she examine her breast during her menstrual period.

B. Tell Mrs. Inwood that the time to examine her breasts is halfway between menstrual periods.

C. Ask Mrs. Inwood if she is doing the breast examination as taught.

D. Examine Mrs. Inwood's breasts.

---

Mrs. Inwood is referred to a physician, who confirms the presence of a mass in her right breast. Mrs. Inwood is admitted to the hospital for a breast biopsy and a possible mastectomy.

---

133. Mrs. Inwood says to the nurse, "My operation is scheduled for tomorrow, but I don't want to lose my breast. Maybe I shouldn't go through with it. What should I do?" Which of these responses should the nurse make first?

A. "The earlier you have the surgery, the better it will be for you."

B. "Can you tell me about what you've been thinking?"

C. "Have you signed the consent form yet?"

D. "Your worries may be unfounded, because your tumor is probably benign."

Mrs. Inwood has a right mastectomy. After a stay in the recovery room, she is brought back to her room. She has an intravenous infusion and a portable suction device (Hemovac) attached to a wound catheter.

134. Mrs. Inwood's right forearm is to be elevated on a pillow. The purpose of this measure is to

A. decrease the risk of hemorrhage.

B. prevent the exudation of fluid from the capillaries.

C. promote the drainage of lymph by gravity.

D. increase the hydrostatic pressure of intercellular fluid.

135. Mrs. Inwood should begin exercises of her right hand and fingers at which of these times?

A. On the first postoperative day.

B. When the intravenous infusion is discontinued.

C. After the Hemovac is removed.

D. As soon as the sutures are taken out.

Mrs. Inwood progresses satisfactorily.

136. The nurse who is changing Mrs. Inwood's dressing observes that Mrs. Inwood, who had previously kept her eyes closed during dressing changes, now has her eyes open but keeps her head turned to the side.

To help Mrs. Inwood to deal with the reality of her body change, the nurse should make which of these statements initially?

A. "When you see your incision, you'll find that it really looks very good."

B. "It is difficult for you to look at your incision the first time."

C. "You're going to have to look at your incision when you go home."

D. "You'll feel better after you have seen your incision."

137. It would be most justifiable to conclude that Mrs. Inwood is beginning to make a positive adaptation to the change in her body image if she were to exhibit which of these behaviors?

A. She refuses assistance in washing her back during morning care.

B. She jokes with the staff members about being lopsided.

C. She tells her husband that she knows she is going to be all right.

D. She consults the nurse about modifications she may need to make in her clothing.

Mr. Harry Stein, 73 years old, has Parkinson's disease. He is to receive care in the clinic. Levodopa (Larodopa) is prescribed for him.

138. Because Mr. Stein has Parkinson's disease, he most probably has which of these symptoms?

   A. Muscle spasms.

   B. Curvature of the spine.

   C. Periodic nocturia.

   D. Drooling.

139. Since Mr. Stein has Parkinson's disease, he most probably has which of these behavioral characteristics?

   A. Euphoria.

   B. Depression.

   C. Overactivity.

   D. Paranoia.

140. Mr. Stein's plan of care should most certainly include which of these goals of care?

   A. To promote independence.

   B. To prevent drug dependence.

   C. To reverse the disease process.

   D. To encourage the use of assistive devices.

141. Mr. Stein should be instructed that the most common early side effect of Larodopa is

   A. diarrhea.

   B. nausea.

   C. frontal headaches.

   D. drowsiness.

Mrs. Barbara Sussman, 54 years old, is admitted to the hospital for a surgical repair of a detached retina in her left eye. She is to receive cyclopentolate hydrochloride (Cyclogyl) eyedrops preoperatively.

142. The nurse should expect Mrs. Sussman to have which of these complaints about the affected eye?

   A. "I can't see with bright lights."

   B. "I see tiny particles floating around in my eye."

   C. "There's a halo around the lights."

   D. "I have sharp pain in my eye."

143. Mrs. Sussman is to receive Cyclogyl eyedrops for which of these purposes?

   A. To dilate the pupil.

   B. To relax the iris.

   C. To reduce intraocular pressure.

   D. To constrict the cornea.

144. Mrs. Sussman is informed that postoperatively she will have a patch covering both eyes. She asks the nurse, "Why will the patch be necessary on my good eye?" To give Mrs. Sussman accurate information, the nurse should give her which of these explanations?

   A. "The pressure in the affected eye will be controlled by resting both eyes."

   B. "Keeping light out of the eyes will contract the ciliary muscles."

   C. "The bleeding in the affected eye will be controlled by applying pressure."

   D. "Decreasing the movement of your eyes will promote healing."

145. In the immediate postoperative period, it
would be most important that Mrs.
Sussman's care plan include which of these
measures?

  A. Encouraging Mrs. Sussman to drink clear
  fluids.

  B. Keeping Mrs. Sussman's head from moving
  suddenly.

  C. Checking Mrs. Sussman's orientation to
  time and place.

  D. Instructing Mrs. Sussman to remain in a
  supine position.

146. Mrs. Unger is to have a determination of
serum levothyroxine ($T_4$) by radioimmuno-
assay. In preparation for the test, Mrs.
Unger should be given which of these
instructions?

  A. "You will need to eat foods high in
  iodine for two days before the test."

  B. "You must get eight hours of sleep the
  night before the test."

  C. "A sample of blood will be drawn from
  you before you leave today."

  D. "An injection of a radioactive drug
  will be given to you."

147. Mrs. Unger asks the nurse, "Why am I
having so much trouble sleeping? How can
that be because of my thyroid problem?"
The nurse's response should include which
of these statements?

  A. "The thyroid gland is unable to control
  the calcium levels that are preventing
  the muscles in your body from relaxing."

  B. "The thyroid gland is attempting to
  compensate for the pituitary gland in
  supplying the hormones needed to
  regulate your biorhythms."

  C. "A decrease of thyroid hormone in your
  body alters nerve impulses."

  D. "An overproduction of thyroid hormone
  causes an acceleration of the metabolic
  rate."

148. Since Mrs. Unger has hyperthyroidism, she
will most probably have which of these
symptoms?

  A. Brittle hair.

  B. Coarse tremors of her hands.

  C. Pallor of her nailbeds.

  D. Palpitations.

149. Mrs. Unger's care plan should give
priority to which of these goals?

  A. To reduce caloric intake.

  B. To minimize sensory stimuli.

  C. To increase muscle strength.

  D. To restore levels of serum calcium.

150. Mrs. Unger should be informed that a common side effect of propylthiouracil is

A. tinnitus.

B. papular rash.

C. anorexia.

D. blurred vision.

151. Lugol's solution is administered to Mrs. Unger for which of these purposes?

A. To minimize the risk of infection in the thyroid gland postoperatively.

B. To stimulate secretion of the antithyroid hormone.

C. To reduce the vascularity of the thyroid gland.

D. To promote visualization of the thyroid gland during surgery.

152. Mrs. Unger should be informed that which of these measures will be carried out postoperatively?

A. Keeping her neck hyperextended.

B. Supporting her head when she moves.

C. Providing her with a straw to drink fluids.

D. Suctioning her oropharynx.

---------------------------------------------

Mrs. Unger has the thyroidectomy as scheduled. When she is brought to her room, she has a dressing over the incision with a wound catheter that is attached to a Hemovac.

---------------------------------------------

153. In the early postoperative period, Mrs. Unger's care plan should give priority to which of these measures?

A. Taking her carotid pulse.

B. Determining her ability to move her head.

C. Monitoring the quality of her voice.

D. Measuring the amount of drainage in her Hemovac.

154. To assess Mrs. Unger for possible hemorrhage, the nurse should take which of these actions?

A. Check Mrs. Unger's ability to swallow.

B. Feel behind Mrs. Unger's neck and shoulders.

C. Palpate the area surrounding Mrs. Unger's dressing.

D. Inspect Mrs. Unger's pharynx.

155. The nurse should assess Mrs. Unger for symptoms of thyroid crisis, which include

A. lethargy.

B. hypotension.

C. cyanosis.

D. hyperpyrexia.

156. The nurse should observe Mrs. Unger for symptoms of hypoparathyroidism, which include

A. muscular twitching.

B. urinary frequency.

C. nausea and vomiting.

D. diplopia.

28

Mr. Martin Eldred, 19 years old, is a college freshman. He is referred to the venereal disease clinic because he has secondary syphilis.

157. Since Mr. Eldred has secondary syphilis, the nurse should expect Mr. Eldred to have which of these lesions?

A. Mucous patches.

B. Gummata.

C. Chancres.

D. Vesicles.

158. In addition to being examined for the presence of lesions, Mr. Eldred should be assessed for which of these symptoms?

A. Urinary frequency.

B. Muscle tremors.

C. Ataxic gait.

D. Sore throat.

159. When interviewing Mr. Eldred, it will be most important for the nurse to achieve which of these goals?

A. To explain Mr. Eldred's treatment plan.

B. To determine Mr. Eldred's attitude about promiscuity.

C. To elicit the names of Mr. Eldred's sexual contacts.

D. To answer questions that Mr. Eldred may have.

160. Mr. Eldred asks the nurse, "What would happen if someone who has syphilis did not receive treatment?" The nurse's response should include the information that the individual may possibly develop which of these complications?

A. Loss of elasticity of cutaneous tissue.

B. Inflammation of blood vessels.

C. Pemphigoid lesions of the skin.

D. Periarteritis nodosa.

161. Mr. Eldred is treated with an antibiotic. Before he leaves the clinic, Mr. Eldred makes all of the following statements. Which one indicates that he needs further instruction about syphilis?

A. "I'm glad that I now have an immunity to this disease."

B. "I didn't think this disease was so serious."

C. "I will certainly have my blood checked regularly."

D. "I will not have sex until my treatment is completed."

Mr. David Orand, 68 years old, is attending the eye clinic for treatment of open-angle glaucoma, which has just been diagnosed. His orders include pilocarpine hydrochloride eyedrops.

162. To prevent an increase in intraocular pressure, Mr. Orand should be given which of these instructions?

A. "Avoid reading the fine print in newspapers."

B. "Limit your television viewing to the nighttime hours."

C. "Avoid straining when you are having a bowel movement."

D. "Drink fluids that are at room temperature."

163. Mr. Orand should be informed that pilocarpine may cause which of these side effects?

A. Drooping of the eyelid.

B. Yellowing of the sclerae.

C. Dryness of the eye.

D. Blurring of vision.

164. Mr. Orand asks the nurse what causes glaucoma. The nurse's response should include the information that which of these physiological defects is present in glaucoma?

A. An increase in the production of aqueous humor.

B. An obstruction of the outflow of aqueous humor.

C. An adhesion of the vitreous humor to the canal of Schlemm.

D. A rise in the tension of the vitreous humor against the anterior chamber.

---

Miss Donna Andrew, 22 years old, is brought to the emergency room. She complains of nausea, vomiting, and abdominal pain.

---

165. When Miss Andrew arrives in the emergency room, the nurse should take which of these actions first?

A. Start an intravenous infusion for Miss Andrew.

B. Ask Miss Andrew to give additional information about her symptoms.

C. Take Miss Andrew's vital signs.

D. Determine when Miss Andrew last ate.

---

The results of diagnostic tests indicate that Miss Andrew has an acute appendicitis. She is admitted to the hospital and scheduled for surgery. Her preoperative orders include meperidine (Demerol) hydrochloride 60 mg.

---

166. Demerol is available in 75 mg. per milliliter of solution. To administer 60 mg. of Demerol to Miss Andrew, the nurse should give how many milliliters of the solution?

A. 0.5

B. 0.8

C. 1.2

D. 1.5

---

Miss Andrew has surgery for a ruptured appendix. A tissue drain is inserted in the wound. Miss Andrew is in stable condition when she is brought to the surgical unit. Her postoperative orders include the administration of meperidine (Demerol) hydrochloride for relief of pain.

---

167. The tissue drain was inserted into Miss Andrew's wound primarily for which of these purposes?

A. To prevent a paralytic ileus.

B. To relieve abdominal pain.

C. To remove purulent matter.

D. To promote healing.

168. Because Miss Andrew had a ruptured appendix, her early postoperative care should give priority to which of these measures?

A. Assessing her for evidence of evisceration.

B. Observing the appearance of her urine.

C. Positioning her on her right side with the head of the bed raised 30 degrees.

D. Administering the prescribed narcotic to her at regular intervals.

169. On Miss Andrew's third postoperative day, she begins to complain of increasing pain in her right lower quadrant. The nurse should take which of these actions first?

A. Ask Miss Andrew if she has passed flatus.

B. Encourage Miss Andrew to walk.

C. Inspect Miss Andrew's incision.

D. Determine when Miss Andrew last had an analgesic.

------------------------------------------------
Mr. Tom Rand, 63 years old, has diagnostic tests that reveal a malignant lesion in the right lung. He is admitted to the hospital for a right pneumonectomy. Following surgery, Mr. Rand is brought to the surgical intensive care unit. He has an intravenous infusion.
------------------------------------------------

170. Mr. Rand's postoperative orders include the administration of an antibiotic. The medication is given primarily for which of these purposes?

A. To treat an existing infection.

B. To hasten healing.

C. To provide prophylaxis.

D. To reduce the number of organisms in the bronchi.

171. When Mr. Rand is returned to his bed, he will be placed in which of these positions?

A. Supine.

B. Low-Fowler's.

C. Side-lying.

D. High-Fowler's.

172. Eight hours after surgery, Mr. Rand's respiratory rate increases and his respirations sound moist. The nurse should take which of these actions first?

A. Check the flow rate of Mr. Rand's intravenous infusion.

B. Auscultate Mr. Rand's chest.

C. Take Mr. Rand's temperature.

D. Assess Mr. Rand for evidence of bleeding.

173. When responding to Mr. Rand's request for medication to relieve his postoperative pain, the nurse assesses the nature of his pain. In addition, which of these assessments will be most important?

A. What is the frequency and amount of his voidings?

B. What is the rate and depth of his respirations?

C. Is he lying in a position of comfort?

D. Is his anxiety level increasing his discomfort?

174. Mr. Rand is to get out of bed to sit in a chair. When assisting him for the first time, it will be most important to take which of these precautions?

A. Keep Mr. Rand from becoming chilled.

B. Administer oxygen to Mr. Rand.

C. Remind Mr. Rand that he may have a change in his center of gravity.

D. Instruct Mr. Rand to elevate the extremity with the intravenous infusion.

------------------------------------------------
Mr. Rand is progressing well, and preparations
are made for his discharge.
------------------------------------------------

175. When Mr. Rand begins to ambulate without
     assistance, emphasis should be placed on
     which of these goals?

     A. To achieve regular bowel elimination.

     B. To develop strength in the muscles of
        the right shoulder.

     C. To adhere to a schedule of self-care
        activities.

     D. To eliminate unnecessary walking as
        much as possible.

------------------------------------------------
Mrs. Martha Massey, 88 years old, is admitted
to the hospital with pneumonia.  Mrs. Massey's
orders include culture and sensitivity studies
of her sputum, a humidifier, oxygen by nasal
cannula p.r.n., and an intravenous infusion.
Her diet order includes food and fluids as
tolerated.
------------------------------------------------

176. On admission, Mrs. Massey is placed in a
     semireclining position.  This measure is
     expected to achieve which of these results?

     A. To promote expansion of Mrs. Massey's
        lungs.

     B. To improve circulation to Mrs. Massey's
        brain.

     C. To relieve pressure on Mrs. Massey's
        sacral area.

     D. To increase Mrs. Massey's venous
        circulation.

177. The culture and sensitivity studies of
     Mrs. Massey's sputum are done for which of
     these purposes?

     A. To determine the number of organisms in
        each cubic millimeter of sputum.

     B. To identify the number of different
        organisms in the sputum.

     C. To select an effective antibiotic.

     D. To eliminate the use of drugs that have
        potential side effects.

178. In addition to using the prescribed
     humidifier, Mrs. Massey would be assisted
     most in raising respiratory secretions by
     which of these measures?

     A. Encouraging her oral intake of fluids.

     B. Teaching her how to splint her chest
        when she coughs.

     C. Changing her position every two hours.

     D. Administering oxygen at regular
        intervals.

179. When assessing Mrs. Massey for early
     symptoms of pulmonary edema, the nurse
     should consider which of these questions?

     A. Has Mrs. Massey's urinary output
        decreased?

     B. Is Mrs. Massey's respiratory rate
        decreasing?

     C. Is Mrs. Massey becoming increasingly
        dyspneic?

     D. Has Mrs. Massey's skin become warm and
        clammy to the touch?

180. Mrs. Massey is to receive skin care every
     four hours.  In the care of her back and
     bony prominences, which of these measures
     should be taken?

     A. Applying alcohol.

     B. Massaging with lanolin lotion.

     C. Washing with soap and water.

     D. Sprinkling cornstarch.

181. The need to change Mrs. Massey's
     intravenous site would most clearly be
     indicated by which of these observations?

     A. Mrs. Massey complains that the
        intravenous infusion is uncomfortable.

     B. The vein used for Mrs. Massey's
        infusion is reddened.

     C. The flow rate of Mrs. Massey's
        intravenous has decreased.

     D. The proximal end of Mrs. Massey's
        intravenous tubing has a streak of
        blood in it.

182. The administration of oxgyen would be indicated if Mrs. Massey developed which of these symptoms in addition to dyspnea?

    A. Elevated body temperature.

    B. Hacking cough.

    C. Increased pulse rate.

    D. Mouth breathing.

----------------------------------------------------

Mr. Mark Ritter, 20 years old, has ulcerative colitis. He is admitted to the hospital because of an exacerbation of his condition.

----------------------------------------------------

183. The nurse should expect Mr. Ritter to state that he has which of these patterns of bowel elimination?

    A. Severe tenesmus followed by tarry stools after each meal.

    B. Frequent, watery stools streaked with mucus and blood.

    C. Alternating diarrhea and constipation.

    D. Strong peristaltic activity preceding evacuation of light-colored, frothy stools.

184. At the time of admission, Mr. Ritter has all of the following problems. Which one should have priority when planning his care?

    A. Anemia.

    B. Dehydration.

    C. Perianal skin irritation.

    D. Electrolyte imbalance.

185. Mr. Ritter is scheduled to have a sigmoidoscopy. After the procedure is done, it will be most important to carry out which of these measures for him?

    A. Cleansing his lower bowel.

    B. Offering him fluids to drink.

    C. Encouraging him to rest.

    D. Taking his blood pressure.

186. Mr. Ritter gives very specific instructions about how to provide care for him. He becomes hostile if his instructions are not followed. When giving care to Mr. Ritter, which of these approaches by the nurse would be most helpful to Mr. Ritter?

    A. Explain the details of a procedure to Mr. Ritter before performing it.

    B. Tell Mr. Ritter that his anger makes it difficult to carry out his care.

    C. Encourage Mr. Ritter to make decisions about his care whenever possible.

    D. Suggest to Mr. Ritter that his methods are not in his own best interest.

----------------------------------------------------

A high-protein, high-vitamin, high-calorie, and low-residue diet is prescribed for Mr. Ritter.

----------------------------------------------------

187. Mr. Ritter refuses to eat most of the food served to him because he thinks the food makes his abdominal cramps worse and increases the number of stools. In attempting to meet Mr. Ritter's nutritional needs, the nurse should take which of these actions?

    A. Explain to Mr. Ritter that his diet order will minimize his symptoms.

    B. Encourage Mr. Ritter to identify his food preferences.

    C. Discuss with Mr. Ritter how the foods ordered for him will coat the ulcerated areas of his bowel.

    D. Have Mr. Ritter's meals liquefied so that he can meet his dietary needs by drinking fluids.

188. The menu includes all of the following desserts. Which one would provide Mr. Ritter with the most protein and calories?

    A. Gelatin with fruit.

    B. Vanilla ice cream.

    C. Custard.

    D. White cake with chocolate frosting.

---
Mr. Ritter does not respond to conservative therapy. He is scheduled to have a total colectomy and ileostomy. In preparation for the surgery, he is to receive total parenteral nutrition (TPN).

---

189. Mr. Ritter's TPN catheter is to be inserted in his right subclavian vein. In preparation for the procedure, Mr. Ritter should be given which of these instructions?

    A. "Your oral intake will be restricted to fluids while you are receiving TPN."

    B. "The TPN catheter will be inserted after you are placed in a sitting position."

    C. "You will be asked to cough during the insertion of the TPN catheter."

    D. "The placement of the tip of the TPN catheter will be checked before feedings are started."

190. The TPN feedings are started for Mr. Ritter. Which of these measures should be added to his daily care plan?

    A. Weighing him at the same time each day.

    B. Determining the pH of his urine after each voiding.

    C. Keeping him on bed rest.

    D. Maintaining him in a semireclining position.

---
Mr. Ritter has a total colectomy and an ileostomy. When his condition is stable, he is brought to his room. He has a disposable ileostomy drainage bag in place. His progress is satisfactory.

---

191. The nurse teaches Mr. Ritter how to change his ileostomy bag. The nurse should explain that it is important that the appliance fit closely around the stoma for which of these purposes?

    A. To prevent the drainage from leaking.

    B. To avoid embarrassing odors from being detected.

    C. To support the underlying tissues.

    D. To protect the mucosa from irritation by fecal matter.

192. To help Mr. Ritter adjust to his ileostomy, which of these suggestions by the nurse would probably be most beneficial for him?

    A. "A member of your family should be taught how to care for the ileostomy."

    B. "Add one new food at a time until you know the effect of each one on your ileostomy drainage."

    C. "Consider joining an organization of persons who have ileostomies."

    D. "Wear loose-fitting clothes that will conceal your ileostomy bag."

---
Mrs. Faith Aronson, 36 years old, is admitted
to the hospital in Addisonian crisis. Her
orders include fludrocortisone (Florinef)
acetate and blood tests.
---

193. On admission, Mrs. Aronson should be
placed in which of these positions?

   A. Semireclining, on her right side.

   B. Flat in bed, with her feet slightly
   elevated.

   C. High-Fowler's, with an overbed table
   placed so that she can rest her arms.

   D. Supine, with her head on a pillow.

194. During the Addisonian crisis, Mrs. Aronson
will have which of these symptoms?

   A. Low blood pressure.

   B. Dyspnea.

   C. Slow pulse rate.

   D. Hypothermia.

195. Mrs. Aronson's initial treatment should be
directed at achieving which of these goals?

   A. To provide a nonstimulating environment.

   B. To restore fluid and electrolyte
   balance.

   C. To control hypermotility of the
   gastrointestinal tract.

   D. To decrease muscle weakness.

196. The results of Mrs. Aronson's blood tests
will report an increased level of which of
these substances?

   A. Sodium.

   B. Glucose.

   C. Potassium.

   D. Chloride.

197. It would be most important that Mrs.
Aronson's care plan include which of these
measures?

   A. Providing minimum care to conserve
   energy.

   B. Encouraging ambulation to prevent joint
   stiffness.

   C. Restricting visitors to reduce exposure
   to infection.

   D. Testing reflexes to detect symptoms of
   nerve involvement.

198. The desired effect of Florinef would be
indicated best by which of these changes
in Mrs. Aronson's condition?

   A. Her food intake is beginning to improve.

   B. She asks to watch television.

   C. Her respirations are 18 per minute.

   D. Her serum sodium level is within normal
   limits.

199. Mrs. Aronson is to continue taking
Florinef after her discharge from the
hospital. She asks, "How long will I have
to take this medication?" Which of these
responses would give her accurate
information?

   A. "The medication will be required until
   you are free of symptoms."

   B. "The doctor will determine the length
   of time you will need to take the
   medication when you are next seen at
   the clinic."

   C. "The medication is usually required for
   a period of two to three months."

   D. "You will be taking the medication in
   varying doses for the rest of your
   life."

200. Before Mrs. Aronson is discharged, she should be given which of the following information about her self-care?

A. Additional medication will be required before she participates in active sports.

B. A prolonged stressful situation may require an increase in the dose of her medication.

C. She should try to limit her intake of salt.

D. She should have a rest period every afternoon.

---

Mr. Frank Barker, 22 years old, is admitted to the hospital following an automobile accident in which he sustained injuries to his abdomen. A ruptured spleen is suspected, and he is scheduled for an emergency exploratory laparotomy. A nasogastric tube is inserted and an intravenous infusion is started.

---

201. During Mr. Barker's preparation for surgery, it would be most important for the nurse to take which of these measures?

A. Monitoring his vital signs every 15 minutes.

B. Keeping his nasogastric tube patent.

C. Counting the flow rate of his intravenous infusion.

D. Teaching him deep-breathing and coughing exercises.

202. The primary purpose of intravenous therapy for Mr. Barker is to

A. replace serum electrolytes.

B. provide access to a vein if a blood transfusion is needed.

C. maintain the volume of circulating body fluid.

D. meet the body's minimum caloric requirement.

---

Mr. Barker has a splenectomy for an extensive laceration of the spleen. Mr. Barker is transferred to the surgical recovery room. He has an intravenous infusion, and a nasogastric tube attached to low, intermittent suction.

---

203. The nurse in the recovery room plans to make all of the following assessments of Mr. Barker. Which one should be made first?

A. The condition of Mr. Barker's surgical dressing.

B. The quality of Mr. Barker's respirations.

C. The type of drainage fom Mr. Barker's nasogastric tube.

D. Mr. Barker's level of consciousness.

---

When Mr. Barker's condition is stable, he is transferred to his room. He makes a rapid recovery. Plans are made for his discharge.

---

204. Mr. Barker says to the nurse, "Why couldn't my spleen be repaired so that it would not have to be removed?" The nurse would be correct in giving Mr. Barker which of these explanations?

A. "The injury to your spleen made it very susceptible to infection, which would spread rapidly through the bloodstream."

B. "The bleeding from an extensive laceration of the spleen cannot be controlled by conservative methods."

C. "The enzymes released by the damaged spleen were beginning to destroy adjacent tissues."

D. "The spleen would have become gangrenous because major blood vessels were severed."

Miss Joan Cannon, 20 years old, is admitted to the hospital for a severe asthmatic attack that did not respond to treatment in the emergency room.

205. During the asthmatic attack, Miss Cannon's respiratory ventilation is altered by which of these pathophysiologic changes?

    A. Atrophy of the bronchial musculature.

    B. Spasms of distended alveoli.

    C. Edema of the bronchioles.

    D. Pulmonary vasoconstriction.

206. Miss Cannon is given isoproterenol (Isuprel) hydrochloride. The desired action of Isuprel for Miss Cannon is to

    A. relax the bronchioles.

    B. constrict the alveoli.

    C. strengthen the intercostal muscles.

    D. suppress neural receptors in the respiratory tract.

Miss Cannon responds to treatment. She is taught to use a nebulizer with Isuprel, and aminophylline suppositories are prescribed. She is discharged and referred to the clinic for further care.

207. The purpose of aminophylline suppositories for Miss Cannon is to

    A. relax the bronchi when she is beginning to have an asthmatic attack.

    B. increase the compliance of her lungs during breathing exercises.

    C. constrict the blood vessels in her respiratory tract when she coughs.

    D. minimize the need for sedation during an attack of asthma.

208. At the first clinic visit, Miss Cannon tells the nurse that she has been using the nebulizer with Isuprel every two to three hours during the day. Excessive use of Isuprel may have which of these effects?

    A. Increased heart rate.

    B. Mental depression.

    C. Constriction of peripheral blood vessels.

    D. Constipation.

209. Miss Cannon says that in the morning when she gets up, she has spasms of coughing and expectorates thick sputum. The nurse should encourage Miss Cannon to follow which of these practices?

    A. Increasing the humidity in her bedroom.

    B. Eating crackers before getting out of bed.

    C. Gargling with an antiseptic solution as soon as she can every morning.

    D. Allowing sufficient time in the morning to avoid being rushed.

Mr. Jack Green, 59 years old, has a cystoscopic examination and biopsy of the bladder. The results confirm that he has cancer of the bladder. The physician explains to Mr. Green that he will need a cystectomy and the surgical construction of an ileal conduit for the drainage of urine. Mr. Green is to receive neomycin sulfate, cathartics, and cleansing enemas for three days preoperatively.

210. The purpose of neomycin for Mr. Green is to

    A. reduce the extent of metastases.

    B. reduce the bacterial count in the intestine.

    C. minimize the number of organisms in the urine.

    D. prevent pulmonary complications.

211. During the first postoperative day, the
     nurse should expect that Mr. Green's urine
     drainage is likely to contain which of
     these substances?

     A. Feces.

     B. Blood.

     C. Bile.

     D. Mucus.

212. Mr. Green should be given which of the
     following instructions about the use of
     his stoma appliance?

     A. "The stoma should be exposed to the air
        daily."

     B. "Empty the drainage collected without
        changing the stoma bag each time."

     C. "The stoma bag should be washed each
        time it is emptied."

     D. "Use an antiseptic solution to cleanse
        the skin around the stoma."

213. It is most important that Mr. Green be
     taught measures that will prevent which of
     these possible consequences of having an
     ileal conduit?

     A. Renal failure.

     B. Kidney stones.

     C. Urinary tract infection.

     D. Uricemia.

214. The nurse performs a physical assessment
     and detects that Miss Wood has enlarged
     cervical nodes.  It would be essential for
     the nurse to obtain which of the following
     data about these nodes?

     A. How many cervical nodes are present?

     B. What is the size of the largest node?

     C. What is the shape of the nodes?

     D. Are the nodes painful to the touch?

215. Miss Wood is suspected of having
     infectious mononucleosis.  The results of
     which of these laboratory tests would
     confirm this diagnosis?

     A. Lymphocyte count.

     B. Hemoglobin.

     C. Blood culture.

     D. Serum amylase.

216. When preparing Miss Wood for the node
     biopsy, the nurse should give her which of
     these explanations of the procedure?

     A. "One or more nodes will be removed
        surgically for examination of cellular
        changes."

     B. "A needle aspiration will remove
        contents of a node for an examination
        that uses a radioactive substance."

     C. "A dye will be injected into a vein to
        allow scanning by an electronic device."

     D. "A heat-detecting apparatus will be
        used to identify abnormal tissue."

217. To control complications of radiation
therapy, which of these measures should be
included in Miss Wood's care plan?

A. Providing meticulous skin care.

B. Encouraging intake of foods high in
protein.

C. Performing passive range-of-motion
exercises.

D. Maintaining a nonstimulating
environment.

218. Miss Wood should be assessed for possible
complications of chemotherapy, which
include

A. cerebral thrombosis.

B. cirrhosis of the liver.

C. infection.

D. visual disturbances.

219. In addition to the symptoms in her joints,
Mrs. Dunn most probably has which of these
alterations in the results of her blood
studies?

A. Increased serum calcium level.

B. Elevated erythrocyte sedimentation rate.

C. Hyperuricemia.

D. Immature thrombocytes.

220. During the acute phase of Mrs. Dunn's
illness, her care plan should include
which of these measures?

A. Putting her involved joints through
full range-of-motion exercises.

B. Massaging her affected joints with
lanolin lotion.

C. Maintaining her joints in a functional
position.

D. Applying elastic bandages to her
weight-bearing joints.

221. When administering aspirin to Mrs. Dunn,
the nurse should take which of these
measures?

A. Check her hearing acuity.

B. Give her 90 ml. of milk.

C. Inspect her oral mucosa.

D. Count her radial pulse.

222. Mrs. Dunn should be informed that Indocin
may have which of these side effects?

A. Photophobia.

B. Orange-colored urine.

C. Gastric distress.

D. Hypotension.

223. Mrs. Dunn's condition improves, and the
physical therapist is teaching her
exercises. Mrs. Dunn should understand
that the primary purpose of exercises for
her is to

A. maintain joint function.

B. halt the progression of the disease.

C. prevent weight gain.

D. reduce joint deformities.

224. Mrs. Dunn says that she enjoys all of the following activities. Which one should she be encouraged to engage in several times a week?

A. Tennis.

B. Swimming.

C. Bowling.

D. Photography.

225. The nurse is discussing health maintenance with Mrs. Dunn. For Mrs. Dunn to live productively, it will be most important for her to have which of these understandings about her condition?

A. Acute episodes will be less severe after menopause.

B. Surgical replacement of joints will be required at a future date.

C. The chronicity of the problem will necessitate alterations in treatment.

D. Loss of the ability to ambulate will be an inevitable occurrence.

--------------------------------------------------
Mr. Herbert Howland, 24 years old, was struck by a car while riding a bicycle. He is admitted to the hospital with an injury of his left knee. There is evidence of bleeding into surrounding tissue, and the knee is painful. X-rays reveal no evidence of fracture. Mr. Howland has a history of sickle cell anemia. Blood tests include the following results: hemoglobin, 7 gm./dl. and hematocrit, 28%. The results of blood gas studies include: $pO_2$, 70 mm. Hg.; $pCO_2$, 38 mm. Hg.; and oxygen saturation, 60%.
--------------------------------------------------

226. When Mr. Howland is admitted, it would be most important for the nurse to take which of these actions?

A. Place a cradle over Mr. Howland's feet.

B. Support Mr. Howland's affected knee in a slightly flexed position.

C. Raise the foot of the bed to elevate Mr. Howland's feet.

D. Assist Mr. Howland into a side-lying position.

227. The nurse should interpret which of these laboratory results as ABNORMAL for Mr. Howland?

A. Hemoglobin, 7 gm./dl.

B. Partial pressure of oxygen, 70 mm. Hg.

C. Erythrocyte sedimentation rate, 80 mm./hr.

D. Hematocrit, 28%.

--------------------------------------------------
Mr. Howland's orders include the application of cold compresses to his affected knee, 2,400 ml. of fluids intravenously every 24 hours, and diet as tolerated.
--------------------------------------------------

228. Mr. Howland asks the nurse why he is receiving fluids intravenously even though he is not in a sickle cell crisis. The nurse's response should include which of the following information about the purpose of this treatment for Mr. Howland?

A. Increasing the volume of body fluids prevents the formation of sickle-shaped blood cells.

B. The administration of parenteral fluids insures an adequate replacement of fluids lost at the site of injury.

C. Supplementing the fluid intake promotes kidney function in order to eliminate the urobilinogen resulting from the destruction of red blood cells in the injured knee.

D. Expanding the blood volume during a period of stress may prevent the onset of clumping of red blood cells.

229. While Mr. Howland is on bed rest, he should be encouraged to perform which of these exercises with his affected leg?

A. Full range of motion.

B. Rotation of the ankle.

C. Flexion and extension of the knee.

D. Extension and dorsiflexion of the foot.

230. For 24 hours after admission, Mr. Howland receives cold compresses to the affected knee. The order is then cancelled. Mr. Howland says that the compresses make him feel better and asks why they are discontinued. The nurse should give him which of these explanations for the discontinuation of the compresses?

A. "The continued use of cold compresses will delay absorption in the knee."

B. "Evidence of continued bleeding in the knee must be established before the cold compresses can be continued."

C. "Ambulation must begin to prevent contractures in the affected knee."

D. "Continued immobilization of the knee will cause the knee joint to fuse."

-------------------------------------------------
Mr. Howland discusses his history of sickle cell anemia with the nurse.
-------------------------------------------------

231. To discuss the genetic transmission of sickle cell anemia, the nurse should have which of these understandings about the genetic factors that pertain to Mr. Howland?

A. He has the autosomal dominant gene for hemoglobin S, which he inherited from one of his grandparents through his parents.

B. He is heterozygous for the sickling gene, which he inherited from his mother.

C. He has the gene for hemoglobin S, which he inherited from the parent who has the sickle cell trait.

D. He is homozygous for the sickling gene, which he inherited from his mother and his father.

232. The results of which of these blood tests were used specifically to establish that Mr. Howland had sickle cell anemia?

A. Hemoglobin electrophoresis.

B. Erythrocyte count.

C. Icterus index.

D. Iron-binding capacity.

-------------------------------------------------
Miss Norma Grey, 26 years old, is admitted to the hospital with infectious hepatitis, Type A.
-------------------------------------------------

233. At the time Miss Grey is admitted to the hospital, it will be most important that the nurse carry out which of these measures first?

A. Obtaining a nursing history from Miss Grey.

B. Identifying Miss Grey's contacts since the onset of symptoms.

C. Assessing Miss Grey's need for medication to relieve pain.

D. Determining whether isolation precautions should be initiated for Miss Grey.

234. When Miss Grey is admitted, she would most probably have which of these complaints?

A. Dyspnea on exertion.

B. Excessive thirst.

C. Anorexia.

D. Eructation.

235. Miss Grey says to the nurse, "I live with my sister and her two children. I'm worried that they may get hepatitis." To respond to Miss Grey's concern, the nurse should give Miss Grey which of the following information about protection against hepatitis?

A. Cortisone preparations may be used to control inflammatory responses to infectious hepatitis.

B. Specific antibiotics may be effective against the virus causing infectious hepatitis.

C. Immune serum globulin may be effective during the incubation period of infectious hepatitis.

D. Prophylactic treatment against infectious hepatitis may be determined by the results of blood cultures of exposed individuals.

236. The nursing care plan for Miss Grey during the acute phase of her illness should give priority to which of these goals?

A. To promote regular bowel elimination.

B. To limit physical activity.

C. To provide mental diversion.

D. To control the antigen-antibody response.

237. Miss Grey's orders include a diet that is high in carbohydrates. Simple carbohydrates should be offered to Miss Grey for which of these purposes?

A. To provide a readily available source of energy.

B. To promote the conversion of protein to glycogen.

C. To increase stores of glucose.

D. To compensate for a decreased tolerance of fats.

238. Miss Grey eats very little breakfast, and at lunch she pushes away her tray without eating. The nurse should take which of these actions?

A. Allow Miss Grey to eat as much or as little as she wishes.

B. Explain to Miss Grey how nutrition will influence the length of her recovery period.

C. Suggest that Miss Grey be placed on total parenteral nutrition therapy.

D. Determine Miss Grey's eating habits before her present illness.

239. A DECREASE in the results of which of these laboratory tests would be most indicative of improvement in Miss Grey's condition?

A. Erythrocyte sedimentation rate.

B. Prothrombin time.

C. Serum glutamic-oxaloacetic transaminase (SGOT).

D. Serum bilirubin.

---------------------------------------------------
Miss Grey's condition improves, and she is being prepared for discharge.
---------------------------------------------------

240. Miss Grey's instruction before discharge should include which of the following information about her self-care during the convalescent period?

A. "Limit your intake of alcoholic beverages to white wine."

B. "Remain on bed rest for the next four weeks."

C. "Avoid eating foods that are highly seasoned."

D. "Resume your physical activity very gradually."

241. Miss Grey would demonstrate a good understanding of the effects of having infectious hepatitis by making which of these statements?

A. "I now have an acquired immunity that will protect me against viral hepatitis."

B. "Having hepatitis means that I cannot be a blood donor."

C. "I will require immunization against hepatitis for the rest of my life."

D. "The permanent liver damage caused by hepatitis has increased the time it takes my blood to clot."

---

The remainder of the questions are individual questions.

---

242. A patient has a hiatus hernia. The treatment should include helping the patient to develop which of these dietary habits?

A. Increasing the intake of complex carbohydrates.

B. Drinking a glass of fluid with meals.

C. Limiting the amount of food eaten at one time.

D. Avoiding foods with a high fiber content.

243. A patient is admitted to the hospital with a complete heart block. In addition to having a slow pulse rate, the patient should be expected to make which of these complaints?

A. "I am dizzy when I sit up."

B. "I have a dull ache under my breastbone."

C. "My feet are swollen at the end of the day."

D. "I have trouble breathing after climbing a flight of stairs."

244. A patient has a kidney transplant. The postoperative orders include the administration of azathioprine (Imuran). The desired effect of Imuran for this patient is to

A. accelerate the production of antibodies.

B. control susceptibility to infection.

C. promote glomerular filtration.

D. prevent rejection of the implanted organ.

245. A patient is admitted to the hospital with bacterial meningitis. The nurse should initiate which of these types of isolation precautions?

A. Respiratory.

B. Enteric.

C. Reverse.

D. Skin.

246. To assess the strength and motor ability of a patient's upper extremities, the nurse should take which of these actions?

A. Instruct the patient to touch the tip of his nose with his forefingers.

B. Observe the patient's ability to raise himself in bed.

C. Have the patient flex and extend his arms.

D. Ask the patient to grasp the nurse's hands simultaneously.

247. A patient is suspected of having pernicious anemia. The nurse should be prepared to assist with which of these diagnostic procedures?

A. Bone marrow aspiration.

B. Complete blood count.

C. Analysis of gastric contents.

D. Gallbladder series.

248. Whenever a patient requests medication for relief of pain postoperatively, which of these nursing actions should be taken first?

A. Determine the time that a medication was last administered.

B. Check the currency of the order for a medication.

C. Assess the patient's need for medication.

D. Consider the level of the patient's threshold for pain.

249. A male patient with severe low back pain is allowed out of bed once daily to go to the bathroom. When carrying out this activity, the patient should be advised to take which of these actions?

A. Keep his head and neck hyperextended.

B. Concentrate on keeping all his muscles relaxed.

C. Take small steps.

D. Avoid any twisting movement of his torso.

250. If a patient with a head injury in the occipital area also has internal injuries that result in hypovolemia, the patient should be maintained in which of these positions?

A. Supine.

B. Semireclining.

C. Side-lying, with the head of the bed elevated 30 degrees.

D. High-Fowler's.

This is the end of the study questions for Nursing Care of Adults. Check to see whether you selected the correct answer to each question by using the answer key on page 45. Explanations for the correct answers in each patient situation begin on page 46. Read the explanations carefully, paying particular attention to the explanations for any questions you answered incorrectly. Then select a reference book from the list of recommended texts on page 71. Read the section that pertains to each patient situation presented in the study questions.

# Answer Key to Study Questions
## for Nursing Care of Adults

| | | | | |
|---|---|---|---|---|
| 1. A | 51. A | 101. C | 151. C | 201. A |
| 2. B | 52. C | 102. D | 152. B | 202. C |
| 3. A | 53. B | 103. C | 153. C | 203. B |
| 4. C | 54. D | 104. B | 154. B | 204. B |
| 5. D | 55. C | 105. D | 155. D | 205. C |
| 6. C | 56. B | 106. C | 156. A | 206. A |
| 7. C | 57. C | 107. C | 157. A | 207. A |
| 8. D | 58. A | 108. B | 158. D | 208. A |
| 9. D | 59. A | 109. A | 159. C | 209. A |
| 10. A | 60. C | 110. A | 160. B | 210. B |
| 11. B | 61. C | 111. D | 161. A | 211. D |
| 12. A | 62. D | 112. C | 162. C | 212. B |
| 13. C | 63. D | 113. A | 163. D | 213. C |
| 14 B | 64. D | 114. B | 164. B | 214. D |
| 15. D | 65. B | 115. D | 165. B | 215. A |
| 16. A | 66. B | 116. D | 166. B | 216. A |
| 17. D | 67. C | 117. C | 167. C | 217. A |
| 18. B | 68. C | 118. B | 168. C | 218. C |
| 19. C | 69. C | 119. A | 169. C | 219. B |
| 20. C | 70. A | 120. A | 170. C | 220. C |
| 21. D | 71. B | 121. C | 171. D | 221. B |
| 22. B | 72. C | 122. D | 172. A | 222. C |
| 23. A | 73. A | 123. B | 173. B | 223. A |
| 24. B | 74. C | 124. A | 174. C | 224. B |
| 25. D | 75. B | 125. C | 175. B | 225. C |
| 26. C | 76. D | 126. D | 176. A | 226. B |
| 27. B | 77. D | 127. C | 177. C | 227. C |
| 28. A | 78. C | 128. A | 178. A | 228. D |
| 29. D | 79. B | 129. A | 179. C | 229. D |
| 30. B | 80. A | 130. D | 180. B | 230. A |
| 31. A | 81. D | 131. C | 181. B | 231. D |
| 32. A | 82. A | 132. D | 182. C | 232. A |
| 33. C | 83. B | 133. B | 183. B | 233. D |
| 34. C | 84. B | 134. C | 184. D | 234. C |
| 35. D | 85. A | 135. A | 185. C | 235. C |
| 36. A | 86. D | 136. B | 186. C | 236. B |
| 37. A | 87. A | 137. D | 187. B | 237. A |
| 38. B | 88. A | 138. D | 188. C | 238. B |
| 39. B | 89. B | 139. B | 189. D | 239. C |
| 40. D | 90. C | 140. A | 190. A | 240. D |
| 41. B | 91. A | 141. B | 191. A | 241. B |
| 42. D | 92. A | 142. B | 192. C | 242. C |
| 43. B | 93. D | 143. A | 193. B | 243. A |
| 44. B | 94. A | 144. D | 194. A | 244. D |
| 45. C | 95. C | 145. B | 195. B | 245. A |
| 46. D | 96. B | 146. C | 196. C | 246. D |
| 47. A | 97. D | 147. D | 197. A | 247. C |
| 48. A | 98. C | 148. D | 198. D | 248. C |
| 49. B | 99. C | 149. B | 199. D | 249. D |
| 50. D | 100. D | 150. B | 200. B | 250. A |

# Explanations for Study Questions
## for Nursing Care of Adults

QUESTIONS 1-12

The onset of pneumonia usually follows an acute viral infection of the respiratory tract. An individual with a history of emphysema has increased susceptibility to pneumonia because of the underlying chronic condition. Bacterial pneumonia, as well as other pneumonias, occur with sufficient frequency that the nurse should have knowledge of causative organisms, symptoms, treatment, and complications as well as nursing measures required for the care of the patient.

Bacterial pneumonia usually starts with a sudden onset of shaking chills, fever, and stabbing chest pain. The patient appears acutely ill. Diagnostic tests include physical examination, chest x-ray, and sputum cultures. Treatment includes antibiotic therapy and measures to improve respiratory function. Oxygen and increased environmental humidity are usually required. The rate of oxygen administration for a patient who has an underlying condition must be considered to prevent narcolepsy. This patient already has an increased arterial partial pressure of carbon dioxide. Therefore, if oxygen is to be administered, the flow rate should not exceed 2 liters per minute.

When the patient has a shaking chill, the patient should be covered with a blanket and kept warm. Temperature should be monitored; high elevations will require measures to reduce the temperature. A high fluid intake is necessary to liquefy secretions and prevent dehydration. Chest physiotherapy will also loosen secretions; removal of secretions will increase the volume of gas exchange in the alveoli. Comfort measures will include assisting the patient into positions of comfort and keeping the patient warm and dry. Treatment will include antibiotic therapy. Medication for relief of chest pain caused by coughing may also be required.

Once the patient's condition begins to improve, copious amounts of sputum will be expectorated. Oral hygiene will be important, especially before food is offered. Encouragement is required to improve the patient's nutritional status. Foods high in protein, such as eggnog, should be offered between meals.

Discharge teaching of the patient should emphasize the importance of preventing respiratory infection. The teaching plan should include urging the patient to avoid contact with persons who have acute symptoms of respiratory infections, to maintain good health habits that include adequate rest and good nutrition, and to report early signs of infection. If the patient smokes, he should be urged to stop.

Follow-up care for any patient with a chronic illness is important. Follow-up care for patients with emphysema includes periodic arterial blood gas analysis. As the vital capacity decreases and the alveolar integrity diminishes, the area available for gas exchange in the lung decreases. The increased carbon dioxide levels and decreased oxygen levels may progress to respiratory acidosis. Symptoms include restlessness and drowsiness.

Waterseal underwater drainage systems are used to re-establish subatmospheric intrapleural pressure to permit lung expansion. Initial symptoms of a pneumothorax include sudden chest pain and dyspnea. The severity of symptoms will depend on the amount of air that enters the pleural cavity. A collapse of the lung may push the heart and large vessels toward the unaffected side and cause disruption in circulation. The trachea shifts and there is an absence of chest movement on the affected side.

## QUESTIONS 13-19

Symptoms of chronic glomerulonephritis are variable. The patient usually appears poorly nourished and has dependent edema. Weakness and fatigability are due to anemia; scheduled rest periods are therefore important for the plan of care.

The procedure for obtaining a clean-catch urine specimen includes cleansing the urinary meatus. The specimen is obtained after the urinary stream has started and the organisms in the urethra have been flushed out. As the glomerular disease progresses, there is accompanying loss of kidney function. The serum creatinine level increases, and other laboratory values are altered. As renal failure develops, the effects on the cardiovascular system increase. When conservative management can no longer maintain fluid and electrolyte balance, dialysis is required to remove fluid and toxic substances normally excreted by the kidneys.

The nursing management of the patient during dialysis includes knowledge of the procedure and possible side effects as well as comfort measures for the patient. The addition of heparin to the dialysate prevents fibrin clots from forming in the drainage tubing. A patient's behavior during dialysis often reflects the patient's fears and anxieties. The nurse should listen for clues in the patient's comments that can be used as a basis for dealing with the concerns expressed by the patient. A patient undergoing dialysis must deal with significant disruption in his/her life. The treatment also imposes changes on the family that require support and understanding by the nurse. The family needs help in understanding the confusion and irritability of the patient before a dialysis treatment, when the symptoms result from the accumulation of waste products in the blood.

QUESTIONS 20-32

The most common cardiac emergency and leading cause of death is a myocardial infarction. A sudden onset of substernal chest pain, unrelieved by rest, that may radiate to the chin, to the arms, or to the epigastrium that results from occlusion of a coronary artery constitutes a life-threatening situation. Immediate assessment of vital signs is required, followed by the administration of a narcotic intravenously for prompt relief of pain in an effort to lower the metabolic rate and reduce oxygen consumption. The patient should be in a semireclining position to promote comfort and respiration. Oxygen may be administered to relieve dyspnea and increase the oxygen supply to the heart.

The initial goals of care for a patient who has a myocardial infarction are to relieve pain, to maintain the cardiac status, and to prevent complications. Constant monitoring of the patient's condition is required. The fear of impending death will cause the patient to be extremely anxious. In addition to remaining with the patient, the nurse should explain what is being done and make the patient feel that he is being competently cared for. The nurse's knowledge and skill are critical in the care of the patient and the family.

It is important for the nurse to have knowledge of the pharmacologic management of a patient with an acute myocardial infarction. Vasodilators, such as Levophed, are administered to improve perfusion of the myocardium. Frequent monitoring of the pulse and blood pressure is required. The pathophysiological alteration resulting from cardiogenic shock includes failure of the left ventricle and tissue hypoxia.

The notification of the family that a member has suffered a myocardial infarction will bring one or more members of the family to the hospital, often in a highly excitable state. The nurse should understand the family's reaction to a sudden, life-threatening situation.

Because the patient's survival requires complete rest and a calm environment, the family should be taken to a quiet area where they will then be informed of the patient's condition. It is essential that the family understand the importance of rest for the patient; visiting should be permitted when the family has control of their behavior.

The management of pain is most important in the care of a patient with a myocardial infarction. The patient's response to medications administered to relieve pain should be noted. When relief of pain is not obtained quickly or when pain recurs before the time that prescribed medication may be given, the physician should be notified immediately. Prescribed narcotics should not be withheld if the patient complains of chest pain. Frequent laboratory studies and monitoring of vital signs provide significant data about the patient's status and this data will be used in determining whether an increase in physical activity should be permitted. The rise in body temperature following a myocardial infarction is an expected reaction of the body to the insult sustained. As soon as the condition is stable, a gradual increase in physical activity is permitted. The prognosis is guarded for a few weeks. Recurrence of chest pain may indicate an extension of the infarction.

Diet prescriptions for a patient following a myocardial infarction most often include a reduction in sodium intake. The nurse should be prepared to instruct the patient about foods highest in sodium, such as whole milk.

Discharge teaching for the patient should include information that will enable the patient to achieve his maximum functioning level.

QUESTIONS 33-39

The use of internal radiation in the treatment of a carcinoma may be determined by the condition of the patient and/or the need to reduce the size of the growth before surgical intervention. The precautions used during radiation therapy include the time spent with the patient, shielding, distance, and the position at which to stand at the bedside to prevent direct exposure to the radiation.

In preparation for internal placement of the radium, the patient receives a cleansing enema. A low-residue diet, including foods such as broiled fish, is prescribed. An indwelling urinary catheter is inserted to prevent displacement of the radium by a distended bladder and to prevent bladder damage by radiation. The patient should understand the importance of maintaining a supine position to prevent dislodgement of the radium.

In preparation for discharge following the radiation treatment, it is important for the patient to understand that once the source of radiation has been removed, no further radiation precautions are required.

The preoperative preparation of the patient for a hysterectomy should include assessment of the patient's emotional readiness for the procedure and providing the needed support, as indicated.

The immediate postoperative care following an abdominal hysterectomy is similar to the care following any surgical procedure. Monitoring of vital signs and observing for evidence of bleeding are important. A hemorrhage would be indicated by a decrease in blood pressure, an increase in pulse rate, and restlessness. Bleeding may or may not be evident. Carrying out of deep-breathing and coughing exercises by the patient following a surgical procedure requiring general anesthesia will prevent pulmonary, vascular, and gastrointestinal complications. The nurse can make the procedure of deep-breathing and coughing easier for the patient by helping the patient support the incisional area. In addition, scheduling the procedure to follow the administration of an analgesic will reduce the patient's discomfort. When a patient has had pelvic surgery, it is particularly important to prevent venous stasis in the lower extremities that may lead to the development of vascular complications. The patient should not sit for extended periods. Ambulation should be encouraged.

## QUESTIONS 40-42

A prolonged inflammatory process with resulting degeneration of liver cells and scarring results in cirrhosis. The pathophysiological alterations develop over a period of time. As liver function decreases, portal hypertension increases and ascites and esophageal varice may develop. Elevated bilirubin levels will lead to pruritis, which requires comfort measures such as bathing with tepid water and applying moisturizing lotion to the skin. To reduce the discomfort caused by ascites, a diuretic is prescribed. The effectiveness of diuretic therapy is best evaluated by weighing the patient daily.

When the underlying cause of the cirrhosis is due to alcohol intake, it is important to observe the patient for continued use of alcohol. When the odor of alcohol is detected on the patient's breath, the patient should be informed of the observation.

## QUESTIONS 43-49

Cataracts most commonly occur past middle age as a result of the aging process. Cataracts may also be congenital, result from trauma, or occur as a complication of diseases that affect the vascular system, such as diabetes mellitus and hypertension. A cataract is the loss of transparency of the crystalline lens or its capsule.

Cataracts cause a gradual loss in vision until the lens becomes completely opaque. The only treatment is surgical removal. The procedure can be done at the convenience of the patient.

When a patient brings any medication to the hospital, it is most important to identify the medication. Newly-admitted patients should always be asked if they brought any medication with them.

Following cataract surgery, measures should be taken to prevent an increase in intraocular pressure. It is most important that the patient be taught to avoid bending over to lift objects from the floor, to prevent sneezing and coughing, and to avoid straining during a bowel movement. If the patient should have nausea, an order for an antiemetic should be obtained. Pain after a cataract extraction is usually slight. Severe pain may be a symptom of hemorrhage and should be reported to the physician without delay.

For the patient who has eyeglasses prescribed, it is important that the patient understand that only the center of the glass will allow clear vision and that the head must be turned to keep objects within the central vision.

A patient with head injury sustained in an accident must be suspected of having injury to the spinal cord. The immediate management of the patient is critical to prevent further damage and loss of neurological function. On arrival in the emergency room, the patient's respiratory function should be assessed first. Monitoring of vital signs should be initiated without delay. Increasing blood pressure and decreasing pulse rate will be indicative of increasing intracranial pressure. The patient's motor and sensory functions should be assessed as soon as possible, and then periodic monitoring is essential to note changes as they may occur. The head and neck should be immobilized. The patient with a head injury must be monitored closely for changes in sensorium. Slurring of speech should be reported without delay. Immediate measures are taken to prevent shock. The plan of care should include measures that will prevent further damage, maintain body functions and prevent complications. Trauma that results in permanent loss of function will require special rehabilitative measures including psychological support.

Once the patient's condition is stable and the condition improves sufficiently for the patient to be allowed out of bed, measures need to be taken to prevent orthostatic hypotension. Measures include raising the head of the bed gradually while monitoring the patient's blood pressure and observing the patient for signs of fainting and shock.

Rheumatic heart disease is the most serious result following acute rheumatic fever. Long-term, conservative management does not always prevent the patient from becoming progressively incapacitated.

In mitral stenosis, the bicuspid valves become calcified and the chordae tendinae become shortened and thickened. Symptoms of mitral stenosis are related to left atrial blood volume and pressure. The back pressure causes left atrial hypertrophy, pulmonary hypertension, and right ventricular hypertrophy. Symptoms usually include fatigue, shortness of breath, pulmonary and peripheral edema, and cyanosis. A cardiac catheterization will provide information about the oxygen concentration and the pressure within the various chambers of the heart.

When a patient expresses intense concern about being in a draft and catching a cold, the most justifiable interpretation is that the patient is dealing with anxiety by means of displacement. The nurse should plan measures that will permit the patient to express concerns about the planned treatment.

The preoperative teaching plan for most patients should include instruction about deep-breathing and coughing exercises. Diaphragmatic breathing and forceful coughing will promote chest expansion and aid in removing pulmonary secretions. The patient should be taught to take several deep breaths and then, before the last expiration, to tighten the abdominal muscles and then cough forcefully.

A chest drainage system is used to remove air and fluid from the chest cavity in order to promote lung expansion and to restore normal gas exchange. Proper maintenance and care of the drainage system is essential to prevent atmospheric air from entering into the system. Measures to maintain the integrity of the waterseal drainage system may include taping the tubing, preventing tension on the tubing that may cause it to become dislodged from the chest, and preventing breakage.

Nursing care of the patient following heart surgery should be reviewed. Measures will include monitoring of vital signs, observing the patient for signs of shock, maintaining fluid and electrolyte balance, measuring intake and output, and relieving pain and discomfort. When the patient is ready, a health teaching program should be started. Progressive activity and regularly scheduled rest periods will be important. Patients anticipate their ability to increase their activity level. Several weeks will be required before the maximum activity level can be determined. A patient's interest in performing specific activities will be determined by their tolerance.

QUESTIONS 61-65

Hyperplasia of the prostate results in a patient's inability to completely empty the bladder. Other symptoms include difficulty in starting a urinary stream, voiding with a smaller stream, terminal dribbling, frequency, urgency, and nocturia. Stasis of urine in the bladder will cause symptoms of cystitis.

Diagnostic evaluation in preparation for the surgical removal of the prostate will include an intravenous pyelogram. Increasing fluid intake following this procedure will promote excretion of the contrast medium used.

Following spinal anesthesia, the patient should be kept in a supine position for several hours. The patient should be well hydrated. Monitoring of the blood pressure is important. The nurse should observe and record the return of sensation and movement of the legs as they occur.

Management of the patient having a prostatectomy should be reviewed. When the patient's condition progresses satisfactorily after surgery, the indwelling urinary catheter is removed. Monitoring of the patient's voiding will be important in determining whether there is urinary retention. Measures to control dribbling should be taught to the patient.

To prevent the possibility of hemorrhage from straining when having a bowel movement, stool softeners, such as Colace, may be prescribed.

## QUESTIONS 66-70

When a patient is brought to the emergency room following a drug overdose, it is most important to identify the drug and amount taken, if possible. Immediate assessment of respirations is required and, when indicated, endotracheal intubation or a tracheostomy is performed to maintain a patent airway. Administration of humidified oxygen may be required. Vital signs are monitored frequently

Cardiac and renal functions are evaluated. Urine, blood, and gastric contents are analyzed to determine drug levels. The level of consciousness is determined and neurological evaluation is performed.

Withdrawal symptoms will include extreme restlessness, and assistance will be required to protect the patient from injury. The patient requires constant attention. Seizure activity may occur. As the patient's consciousness returns, the patient should be oriented to being in the hospital and attended by a nurse. Patience in giving emotional support will be most important when the patient recovers sufficiently and begins to display agitated and aggressive behavior. It is important to remain quietly with the patient and permit the patient to express feelings. At the appropriate time, the patient should be encouraged to participate in a therapy program.

## QUESTIONS 71-74

A patient with a peptic ulcer has a history of epigastric pain relieved by eating. A gastroscopy provides direct visualization of the ulcerated area and permits a biopsy of tissue. Sedation and topical anesthesia are administered before the gastroscope is passed through the mouth into the stomach. Following the procedure the patient is given nothing by mouth until the gag reflex returns.

Recurrent ulcers that do not respond to medical therapy require surgical removal of the ulcerated area. Drainage from the nasogastric tube should be dark red for about twelve hours after surgery. Care of the nares should include cleansing with a swab moistened with water and then applying a water-soluble lubricant. Care of the patient should include measures to prevent pulmonary complications, monitoring intake of parenteral fluids, monitoring vital signs, and relieving incisional pain.

Instructions before the patient is discharged should include information about diet to meet nutritional needs. Depending on the extent of the resection, hematinics may be prescribed to supplement nutritional deficiencies. It is important to inform the patient about the possible development of the dumping syndrome. Early symptoms include weakness, faintness, and dizziness. The patient should be instructed to reduce intake of simple carbohydrates, to avoid fluids with meals, and to lie down after eating to delay emptying of the stomach.

QUESTIONS 75-79

The emergency treatment of a patient who has

sustained burns will depend on the cause of the burns, the condition of the patient, the extent of the burned areas, and the depth of the burns. As soon as the patency of the airway is established, attention is given to the prevention of shock. Morphine sulfate is administered intravenously to hasten absorption of the drug. Oliguria develops when circulating fluid volume is not maintained; the shock is reflected in a decreasing blood pressure. Maintaining the rapid flow rate prescribed for intravenous fluids is essential. The development of renal failure will be indicated by an average hourly urine output of less than 30 milliliters.

The exposure method of treating burns is used to control bacterial growth. The nursing management of a patient with burns should be reviewed. Meeting the patient's physical and psychological needs through the rehabilitative stage is important.

QUESTIONS 80-82

Transient cerebral ischemia causes sudden, temporary loss of cerebral function. The symptoms of motor, sensory, or visual loss depend on the area affected by the temporary ischemia. Persons who experience confusion, vertigo, and muscular weakness temporarily are having attacks of transient cerebral eschemia and are at high risk to have a stroke. These symptoms require that measures be taken to prevent injury to the patient if an attack occurs while the patient is out of bed. A carotid angiogram is done to determine the presence of an obstruction in blood vessels within the brain. Other diagnostic tests include computerized tomography. Treatment may include drug therapy and surgical intervention.

QUESTIONS 83-89

There is a high incidence of hip fractures in the elderly. Skin traction is often applied temporarily to immobilize the extremity, to reduce muscle spasms, and to relieve pain. The skin of the affected extremity should be inspected for intactness and circulatory adequacy. Measures should be taken to prevent breakdown of the skin. It is important to explain to the patient the pulling sensation that will be caused by the traction. Traction apparatus should be checked to maintain proper function.

Attention should be given to the behavior of the patient. The patient may experience varying degrees of anxiety about what is happening. The shock of the trauma may cause the patient to become confused and disoriented.

To prevent complications caused by immobility, surgical intervention should be carried out as soon as the patient's condition has been assessed. Following surgery, the affected extremity should be maintained in a slightly abducted position. The patient should be encouraged to dorsiflex and extend the foot. Turning is usually permitted onto the unaffected side. A pillow is placed between the legs to maintain the affected leg in correct alignment.

Monitoring of the intravenous fluids administered to an elderly person is essential to detect symptoms of fluid overload. Moist respirations and the onset of dyspnea require that the flow rate of the intravenous infusion be decreased.

When quadriceps-setting exercises are prescribed in preparation for ambulation, the patient should be instructed to lie in a supine position, press the back of the knee against the bed, and attempt to lift the heel.

QUESTIONS 90-98

Diabetes mellitus is the result of the body's inability to produce or utilize insulin. Review of symptoms, diagnostic tests, and management of insulin-dependent and non-insulin-dependent diabetes is important.

Each patient requires a teaching plan. After establishing the patient's readiness to learn, the nurse should determine what the patient knows about diabetes. The teaching plan should include teaching measures that will control the diabetes and prevent or minimize the development of complications. It is important for the patient to understand the need to ingest a carbohydrate before strenuous exercise in order to avoid having a hypo-glycemic reaction. Symptoms of hypoglycemia, such as feeling tremulous, will enable patients to take appropriate action without delay. The patient's use of the food exchange list should include the ability to make appropriate food exchanges, such as exchanging bread for white rice or an egg for a serving of tuna fish.

When teaching self-administration of insulin, the nurse should explain the action of insulin. Understanding that the peak action of insulin occurs in the late afternoon will prepare the patient to eat a snack before a hypoglycemic reaction occurs.

Causes of ketoacidosis include infections. Results of blood tests will reveal the hydrogen ion concentration to be increased, the pH decreased, the serum bicarbonate and the serum potassium levels low. Serum carbon dioxide levels will provide information about the patient's buffering system. The patient's response to treatment will include evaluating blood test results. As blood chemistries show results approaching normal, an intravenous infusion of glucose will be prescribed to prevent the development of hypoglycemia.

QUESTIONS 99-109

A person with hypertension has a sustained systolic blood pressure above 150 mm. Hg. and a diastolic blood pressure above 90 mm. Hg. Hypertension, usually detected on routine physical examination, is often free of symptoms, but it is the major cause of heart failure, stroke, and renal disease. When symptoms are present, they usually include morning headaches, fatigability, and feelings of nervousness and irritability. Hypertension is related to the loss of elasticity in the arterioles. Vasoconstrictor stimuli that affect the response of blood vessels include stress, caffeine, tobacco, and obesity.

Treatment of hypertension is directed toward keeping weight within normal limits, limiting use of stimulants, identifying stressful situations, lowering cholesterol levels, reducing intake of salt, and treating any underlying physical conditions.

Patient education about restricting sodium in the diet should include information about foods high in sodium, including substances used to flavor foods, such as soy sauce. The instruction should also include information on the importance of reading the labels on prepared foods.

Loss of the contractability of the heart that is necessary to maintain adequate cardiac output leads to congestive heart failure. Increased pulmonary venous pressure causes transudation of fluid from pulmonary capillaries. The patient will have symptoms of dyspnea and a moist cough. Increased systemic venous pressure causes dependent edema. Bed rest will reduce the workload of the heart, and positioning the patient in a semireclining position will improve respiratory efforts. Since edematous tissue is prone to the development of decubiti, it is most important to change the patient's position frequently. Bed rest will cause fluid shift to the sacral areas, so careful attention should be given to maintaining tissue integrity in this area. Lanoxin is administered to increase the force and efficiency of the myocardium. To administer Lanoxin 0.5 mg. when the dosage available is 0.25 mg. tablets, the nurse should administer two tablets. Loss of appetite may be an early indication of a side effect of Lanoxin. The desired therapeutic effect of Lanoxin will be noted in the improved quality of the pulse. The desired therapeutic effect of Lasix is to eliminate the excessive accumulation of body fluid. The desired effect would be best indicated by the patient's weight loss. The use of diuretics may lead to a depletion of potassium; foods high in potassium should therefore be served. Complications of hypokalemia include the development of arrhythmia.

QUESTIONS 110-115

The major symptoms of peripheral arterial disease include intermittent claudication relieved by rest and decreased or absent peripheral pulses in the feet. When obtaining a nursing history, the nurse should ask the patient how far he can walk without discomfort. An assessment of the patient's lower extremities will reveal that the feet feel cold to the touch, that there is an absence of hair, and that pulses are diminished or absent.

When surgery is planned, an arteriogram is performed to confirm the diagnosis and to identify more accurately the site of obstruction.

The use of a contrast medium for the test necessitates determining whether the patient has a history of allergies.

Tissue ischemia related to poor oxygen transport is the nursing diagnosis upon which the patient's care should be based. Measures should include meticulous foot care and daily inspection of the extremities to detect signs of injury.

Following a femoral bypass graft, measures in the patient's care should include monitoring peripheral pulses, noting the color and temperature of the feet, and preventing the patient from assuming positions that require sharp flexion of joints. Intravenous fluids are usually administered until the patient's blood pressure is approximately the same as his preoperative blood pressure.

QUESTIONS 116-122

The nurse should interpret the blood test results in question #116 as abnormal findings. Laboratory reports usually include the normal range for blood values, but a nurse should know the normal range for routine blood tests. Abnormal blood test results may indicate the need for further diagnostic tests, which in this situation include a bone marrow aspiration.

When a patient expresses anxiety about having a diagnostic procedure, it is important for the nurse to determine what it is about the procedure that is of concern. Usually the only preparation of the patient that is required for a bone marrow aspiration is a careful explanation of the procedure. It is essential that the patient sign an informed consent for the procedure.

The initial plan of care for a patient who has leukemia should give priority to conserving the patient's energy. Side effects of chemotherapy include the development of stomatitis. A mild alkaline solution should be used to rinse the mouth. Chemotherapy depresses a patent's immunological defense mechanism; the patient should therefore avoid sources of infection, which include crowds. Because of the patient's increased suscepti- bility to infection, symptoms of chills and fever should be reported without delay.

QUESTIONS 123-125

Intrinsic cancer of the larynx involves the vocal cords. An early symptom is hoarseness, because the tumor interferes with the proxima- tion of vocal cords when speaking. The diagnostic test used to confirm the presence of the cancer is a direct laryngoscopy with tissue biopsy.

When a patient makes a statement that members of the family have died from cancer, the nurse should encourage the patient to continue to talk so that his concerns may be more accurately determined.

Since the surgical procedure will prohibit the patient from speaking, the preoperative preparation for the patient should include establishing a method of communication to use postoperatively.

Postoperatively, the patient with a laryngectomy tube in place will require frequent suctioning. Suction should be applied only when the catheter is being removed.

## QUESTIONS 126-128

A patient who is in a coma following a cerebrovascular accident is prone to many complications. The complication that poses an early risk is an acute upper respiratory infection. To prevent the development of contractures and to promote circulation, priority should be given to performing passive range-of motion exercises. When the patient's treatment includes nasogastric tube feedings, the rate of flow should be slow to prevent aspiration from regurgitation.

The care of a patient who has a cerebovascular accident requires many supportive and preventive measures during the acute stage of the illness as well as through the convalescent and rehabilitative period. It is important to review the care of a patient who has a cerebrovascular accident.

## QUESTIONS 129-137

Based on established guidelines for hypertension, it would be important in this situation to have the patient rest for about 20 minutes and then to retake the blood pressure.

An important principle of teaching that should be applied to health care teaching is that after assessing the patient's readiness to learn, the nurse should ascertain what the patient already knows. To examine the medial half of the left breast, the left hand should be placed under the head. This procedure will tense the pectoral muscles to provide a flatter surface against which to palpate. There are normal changes that occur in the breast around the time of the menstrual period, but the nurse should examine a patient's breast when informed that a lump was felt during self-examination. By performing the breast examination in this situation, the nurse can determine whether a lump is present, and at the same time help to allay the patient's fears if no lump is felt.

Several diagnostic procedures are available to confirm the presence of a lump in the breast. The diagnosis of cancer in the breast can be confirmed only by a pathological examination of tissue obtained by biopsy. When a woman is admitted to the hospital because of a questionable lump in the breast, there is always a real fear of having cancer. When a patient expresses this concern, the nurse should attempt to obtain information from the patient about the implications perceived by the patient.

The care of a patient following a mastectomy should be reviewed. The arm on the affected side may be elevated to prevent edema by promoting drainage of lymph by gravity. An exercise program should be initiated as soon after surgery as possible. The exercise may begin with the opening and closing of the fist; but within 24 hours, active exercise of the entire arm should be encouraged. A goal of care in the postoperative period is to assist the patient in dealing with the alteration in body image. If the patient is unable to look at the surgical site, it is appropriate for the nurse to acknowledge the patient's difficulty. This demonstrates understanding and acceptance of the patient's problem. Positive adaptation to the change in body image will begin when the patient begins to make plans to resume her former life style and considers the adjustments, if any, that will be required in her clothing and activities.

QUESTIONS 138-141

Early symptoms of Parkinson's disease include stiffening of joints, muscular rigidity, tremors that begin in one hand, and difficulty in motor activities. As the condition progresses, the patient develops a stooped posture, drooling, and a masklike expression. Patients with Parkinson's disease frequently have signs of depression. An important goal of care is to promote the patient's independence. Laradopa is administered in increasing doses to control symptoms of the disease. Side effects of the drug include nausea, vomiting, anorexia, and hypotension.

QUESTIONS 142-145

A retinal detachment is a partial or complete separation of the sensory layer from the epithelial layer. The separation may be caused by trauma or degenerative changes. The symptoms appear suddenly and include seeing flashes of light, particles floating in the eye, a sensation of a veil in front of the eye, and finally loss of vision.

Preoperatively, Cyclogyl is administered to dilate the pupil. It is important to explain to the patient preoperatively the activities she will be permitted in the early post-operative period. When both eyes will be covered, the patient should be informed that use of the unaffected eye will cause movement of the affected eye. To promote healing, movement in the affected eye will be decreased by covering both eyes. In the postoperative care of the patient, it is most important to prevent sudden movements of the head and to avoid activity that may increase intraocular pressure.

## QUESTIONS 146-156

Early symptoms of hyperthyroidism usually include feelings of nervousness, palpitations, and sleeplessness. These symptoms are caused by an overproduction of thyroid hormone, which increases the metabolic rate. Several diagnostic tests are available, and the nurse should be prepared to give the patient an explanation of the tests to be performed. A $T_4$ is a test performed on a sample of the patient's blood without any previous preparation of the patient.

An important goal of care for a patient with hyperthyroidism is to promote rest by mini-mizing all external stimuli. Propylthiouracil is administered to produce an euthroid state

An occasional side effect is a papular rash. If the patient develops any sign of infection, she may be required to stop the medication. When surgical removal of the thyroid is indicated, Lugol's solution may be prescribed for the patient to reduce the vascularity of the thyroid gland.

Preoperatively the patient should be informed that her head will be supported when she is moved. The neck should not be hyper-extended or flexed. In the early postoperative period it is important to monitor vital signs and to observe for signs of bleeding. Because blood will drain by gravity, it is important to feel behind the patient's neck and shoulders. Deep breathing is encouraged, but coughing should be avoided for the first two days. Possible laryngeal nerve damage is assessed during the first 24 hours by monitoring the quality of the patient's voice. The patient should be observed for symptoms of an impending thyroid crisis, which include hyperpyrexia and tachycardia. If a euthyroid state was achieved before surgery, it is unlikely that the patient will have this complication. Assessment of the patient for symptoms of hypoparathyroidism should include observing for signs of muscular twitching, tingling sensation in the fingers and toes, and carpopedal spasms. If symptoms of hypoparathyroidism develop, calcium gluconate for intravenous administration should be readily available.

## QUESTIONS 157-161

A patient with secondary syphilis will have macular, papular, or papulosquamous lesions on the skin. Mucous patches also occur on the genital, perineal, and oropharyngeal areas. Additional symptoms include sore throat, headache, malaise, and enlarged lymph nodes. It is important to elicit the names of sexual contacts in order to prevent further spread of the disease. Persons with untreated syphilis develop inflammation of blood vessels, as well as complications affecting the nervous system, heart, and bone. It is important that the patient understand that infections do reoccur and that immunity does not follow after having had the disease and treatment.

## QUESTIONS 162-164

Treatment for glaucoma is directed at decreasing the elevated intraocular pressure that is caused by an obstruction of the outflow of aqueous humor. The patient should be instructed to avoid activities that increase intraocular pressure, such as straining when having a bowel movement. A stool softener may be prescribed for patients with constipation.

A frequent side effect of pilocarpine is temporary blurring of vision.

## QUESTIONS 165-169

When a patient complains of nausea, vomiting, and abdominal pain, it is important to obtain further information about the symptoms, such as the description and location of the pain.

Once the diagnosis of acute appendicitis is made and the patient is scheduled for surgery, there may be limited time for the preoperative preparations. It is important to determine the time the patient last ate and to keep the patient fasting. Baseline data should be obtained and explanations should be given to the patient about the proposed surgery.

To administer 60 mg. of Demerol that is available in 75 mg. per milliliter of solution, the nurse should give 0.8 milliliters.

When a tissue drain is inserted in the surgical wound, the purpose is to permit drainage. To promote localization of the infected site of the appendix, the patient should be maintained in a semireclining position on the right side or on the back. The patient usually improves rapidly, and ambulates and manages self-care independently. If the patient begins to complain of increasing abdominal pain on the third postoperative day, the nurse should inspect the surgical incision for evidence of an infection.

muscles of the shoulder.

QUESTIONS 170-175

A pneumonectomy is performed when a less radical procedure is not possible to remove the diseased portion of the lung. Antibiotic therapy postoperatively is prescribed to provide prophylaxis. To provide for maximum expansion of remaining lung tissue, the patient shold be kept in a high-Fowler's position. If the patient is unable to tolerate a sitting position, lower elevations of the head of the bed are permitted. During the early postoperative period, it is essential to closely monitor vital signs and to monitor blood gases. Frequent assessment of respiratory rate, depth, and quality is important in detecting early signs of fluid overload that will require slowing the intravenous flow rate. Before administering medication for relief of pain, the nurse should assess the rate and depth of respirations.

Since a pneumonectomy involves a radical dissection, it is important to inform the patient when getting him out of bed that he may have a change in his center of gravity that will affect his balance.

As soon as possible after surgery, the patient should be taught exercises of the arm and shoulder on the affected side in order to maintain posture and to regain strength in the

QUESTIONS 176-182

On admission to the hospital, a patient with pneumonia should be supported in a semi-reclining position to promote expansion of the lungs. To relieve pain, the patient may wish to be turned onto the affected side to splint the area.

Before antibiotic therapy is started, culture and sensitivity studies of the patient's sputum are done to select the most effective antibiotic for the causative organism. Removal of respiratory secretions will be facilitated when oral intake of fluids is sufficient to liquefy secretions.

Elderly persons who probably have a compromised cardiovascular system should be observed for fluid overload by assessing their respirations for signs of dyspnea. Dyspnea and an increased pulse rate may also indicate that the patient should have oxygen administered.

To maintain skin integrity, the patient's position should be changed frequently, the skin should be kept clean and dry, and pressure areas should be massaged lightly with lanolin lotion.

The development of a phlebitis would be

clearly indicated if the site over the vein used for the intravenous infusion became reddened.

## QUESTIONS 183-192

A patient with ulcerative colitis has frequent, watery stools that are streaked with mucus and blood. As a result of an acute exacerbation of the symptoms, priority must be given to the patient's electrolyte imbalance. To evaluate the current status of the disease, the patient is scheduled for diagnostic examinations that may include a sigmoidoscopy and a barium enema. When preparing the patient for these procedures, cathartics are contra-indicated. Following the procedure, the patient should be given an opportunity to rest.

The psychological aspects of care for a patient with ulcerative colitis require special attention. The patient often displays a wide range of psychological symptoms. If the patient gives specific instructions about how to provide care for him and if he becomes hostile when his instructions are not followed, the nurse should encourage the patient, when-ever possible, to make decisions about his care.

Meeting the nutritional needs of a patient with ulcerative colitis is a challenge. Any foods that cause distress should be avoided.

The patient should be encouraged to identify food preferences and his requests should be met, if at all possible. Of the choices of desserts offered in question 188, custard would provide the most protein and calories.

The preoperative preparation of a patient for a total colectomy usually requires intensive fluid, blood, and protein replacement. Total parenteral nutrition is often used to provide the patient with the caloric intake required. In preparation for inserting the TPN catheter into the right subclavian vein, the patient should be informed that the position of the tip of the catheter will be checked by x-ray. To assess the effectiveness of the TPN feedings, the patient should be weighed at the same time daily.

During the recuperative phase following an ileostomy, the patient should be involved in his self-care, and explanations should be given to him for measures taken by the nurse. A closely fitting appliance is important to prevent drainage from leaking and to prevent excoriation of the skin surrounding the stoma.

To help the patient adjust to the ileostomy, it would be important that the patient consider joining an organization of persons who have ileostomies.

## QUESTIONS 193-200

A patient in Addisonian crisis is acutely ill and in shock. The patient should be placed in a supine position without a pillow, and with the feet slightly elevated. Symptoms of an Addisonian crisis include shock, rapid respiration, low blood pressure, rapid pulse, fever, pallor, and extreme apprehension. The initial treatment is directed at restoring fluid and electrolyte balance. The results of blood tests will reveal elevated serum level of potassium and decreased levels of serum sodium and glucose.

It is essential that during the early treatment every effort be made to conserve the patient's energy. Care is given to meet essential needs only. Any overexertion by the patient may lead to circulatory collapse. An early indication that the Florinef was achieving the expected therapeutic effect would be blood test results showing that the serum sodium level was within the normal range.

Before the patient is discharged, it will be most important that the patient understands that Florinef will be required in varying doses for the rest of the patient's life. Situations that will alter the patient's dose of medica- tion should be made clear so that the patient will know how to adjust the medication in times of stress.

## QUESTIONS 201-204

A splenectomy following trauma is an emergency procedure. Diagnosis and preparation for surgery must be done quickly. Monitoring of vital signs every 15 minutes, or even more frequently, is essential. The primary purpose of intravenous fluids is to maintain the volume of circulating fluids. Blood transfusions are often required.

Following any surgical procedure, the assessment of respirations should be made first.

Emergency procedures, such as a splenectomy, do not afford time to teach the patient preoperatively. The detailed explanations must be made after the surgery has been performed. Severe lacerations or excessive bleeding in the spleen cannot be controlled by conservative methods because the spleen is too vascular to respond quickly enough to save the patient from hemorrhaging to death.

## QUESTIONS 205-209

Prolonged attacks of asthma often require hospitalization. The patient usually has a history of hypersensitivity to a known substance. The obstruction to respirations is edema of the passages of the respiratory tract. Isuprel is administered to relax the bronchioles. A nurse should be familiar with the variety of drugs used to treat patients with acute asthma. The patient requires frequent assessment to detect side effects. The state of the patient's anxiety during an attack requires constant attention and a calm, reassuring approach.

Aminophylline suppositories are prescribed for the patient to use at the onset of an asthmatic attack to relax the bronchi. Patients should be cautioned that excessive use of drugs that are used in the treatment of asthma will increase the heart rate.

To facilitate the removal of thick respiratory secretions, the patient should be instructed to liquefy secretions by increasing environmental humidity and maintaining a high intake of fluids.

## QUESTIONS 210-213

The preoperative preparation of a patient scheduled for a cystectomy includes the administration of neomycin to reduce bacterial count in the intestinal tract.

Postoperatively, the urine drainage from the ileal conduit should be straw colored and contain mucus that is sloughing from the intestinal lining.

Initially, a temporary stoma appliance is used; it remains in place as long as it is intact. The drainage can be emptied without removing the bag. It is most important that the patient maintain a high fluid intake to prevent urinary tract infections. Careful emptying of the conduit will also prevent urinary stasis, which could lead to a urinary tract infection.

## QUESTIONS 214-218

When assessing a patient for the presence of palpable nodes, the nurse should note their location, the size of all the nodes felt, the consistency of the nodes, whether they are freely movable, and whether they are tender or painful to the touch.

A patient with infectious mononucleosis would have an elevated lymphocyte count that has atypical lymphocytes.

When Hodgkin's disease is suspected, one or more nodes will be removed surgically and examined for a large atypical tumor cell, called the Reed-Sternberg cell. Identification of the tumor cell is followed by an attempt to locate the sites at which the cells are present. Treatment is determined by the sites involved. Radiation is one of the methods used in the treatment of the disease. Complications of radiation therapy can usually be controlled by providing meticulous skin care. While a patient is receiving chemotherapy, frequent assessment for signs of an infection should be made.

## QUESTIONS 219-225

A patient with acute rheumatoid arthritis will have leukocytosis and an elevated erythrocyte sedimentation rate.

When the joints are acutely inflamed, they should be supported in a functional position. When anti-inflammatory drugs, such as aspirin, are administered for relief of pain, they should be taken with milk to prevent gastric irritation. When Indocin is prescribed, the patient should be informed that this drug may cause gastric distress and that the side effects can be minimized by taking the drug with food.

When a patient with rheumatoid arthritis is receiving instruction about exercise, it is most important that the patient understand that the purpose of the exercises is to preserve joint function and to prevent deformities.

Swimming is the exercise that a patient should be encouraged to perform regularly because it exercises all the muscles in the body while water supports the joints.

For a patient with rheumatoid arthritis to live productively, it is important that the patient understand that the chronicity of the condition will necessitate alterations in treatment.

## QUESTIONS 226-232

Any individual who sustains an injury to a body part will have swelling, bleeding, pain, and loss of function of the affected part. nitial treatment includes immobilizing the part in a functional position.

A patient who has a history of sickle cell anemia will have a low hemoglobin, a low hematocrit, and a decreased partial pressure of oxygen. When this patient sustains a traumatic injury to a joint, he will be vulnerable to hypoxic damage caused by the sickling process. Immediate preventive measures include the administration of intravenous fluids in an effort to expand the blood volume and prevent the onset of clumping of red blood cells. While the knee is immobilized, the only exercise the patient should perform is dorsiflexion and extension of the foot.

The application of cold compresses to a joint to control bleeding should be used judiciously and discontinued as soon as possible to permit absorption in the knee. The extended use of cold compresses also has the danger of precipitating the onset of sickling in a patient wih sickle cell anemia.

A patient with sickle cell anemia is homozygous for the sickling gene, which was inherited from both parents. To determine whether the patient has sickle cell anemia or sickle cell trait, a hemoglobin electrophoresis must be done. A patient with a sickle cell trait will have a normal hemoglobin and a normal hematocrit. This person has the hemoglobin A in his cells that ordinarily prevents them from sickling.

## QUESTIONS 233-241

At the time a patient with hepatitis is admitted to the hospital, it is important to determine whether isolation precautions should be initiated to control spread of the disease.

Immune serum globulin may be effective during the incubation period of infectious hepatitis.

During the acute phase of the illness, the patient will have complaints of anorexia and fatigue. Treatment will include bed rest to limit the patient's physical activity. Offering the patient simple carbohydrates will provide a readily available source of energy. It is important to encourage the patient to eat and to help the patient understand that nutrition will influence the length of the recovery period from the illness. The elevation of serum transaminase will reflect the extent of liver tissue damaged; a decrease of this laboratory value is most indicative that the condition of liver cells has improved. Following a period of bed rest, a gradual increase in activity level is permitted. Scheduled rest periods continue to be important for several weeks. A patient with a history of hepatitis should not be a blood donor.

## INDIVIDUAL QUESTIONS 242-250

242. A hiatus hernia occurs when the cardiac portion of the stomach extends into the thorax because of an enlarged opening in the diaphragm. Conservative treatment includes the use of antacids, sitting up after a meal, and limiting the amount of food eaten at one time.

243. A failure in the conduction system of the heart will result in heart block. The heart rate is slowed and cardiac output

is decreased. The decreased cardiac output will cause the patient to become dizzy when sitting up or it may cause fainting.

244. The administration of Imuran to a patient following a kidney transplant is expected to prevent rejection of the implanted organ.

245. The organism causing bacterial meningitis enters the body through the nose and mouth by the droplet method. Respiratory precautions are required during the acute phase of the illness.

246. Assessment of a patient's muscle strength is best accomplished by determining the patient's ability to flex or extend an extremity against resistance. Asking the patient to grasp the nurse's hands simultaneously will provide data comparing the equality of strength of both of the patient's upper extremities.

247. A patient suspected of having pernicious anemia will have a gastric analysis to determine the volume of hydrochloric acid present. A Schilling test may also be performed to determine the patient's ability to absorb oral vitamin $B_{12}$.

248. Whenever a patient requests medication for relief of pain, the nurse should first assess the patient's need for medication. If the currency of an order or the time that the medication was last given does not permit administration of a medication, the nurse should consult with the physician about the patient's complaint of pain.

249. Health teaching for a patient with low back pain must include the need to avoid any twisting movement of the torso to prevent muscle strain.

250. Generally, a patient with a head injury in the occipital area will be maintained in a supine position to lower cerebral venous pressure. A patient wih a supratentorial head injury may be placed in a semi-reclining position, depending on the level of intracranial pressure.

# References for Nursing Care of Adults

Billings, Diane McGovern, and Lillian Gatlin Stokes. Medical-Surgical Nursing. St. Louis, MO: The C. V. Mosby Co., 1982.

Brunner, Lillian Sholtis, and Doris Smith Suddarth. Textbook of Medical-Surgical Nursing, 5th ed. Philadelphia: J. B. Lippincott Co., 1984.

Gilman, Alfred Goodman, et al. The Pharmacological Basis of Therapeutics, 6th ed. New York: Macmillan Publishing Co., 1980.

Jones, Dorothy A., et al. Medical-Surgical Nursing - A Conceptual Approach, 2nd ed. New York: McGraw-Hill Book Co., 1982.

Krause, Marie V., and Kathleen L. Mahan. Food, Nutrition and Diet Therapy, 7th ed. Philadelphia: W. B. Saunders Co., 1984.

Lewis, Sharon Mantik, and Idolia Cox Collier. Medical-Surgical Nursing: Assessment and Management of Clinical Problems. New York: McGraw-Hill Book Co., 1983.

Phipps, Wilma J. et al. Shafer's Medical-Surgical Nursing, 7th ed. St. Louis, MO: The C. V. Mosby Co., 1980.

Rodman, Morton J. and Dorothy W. Smith. Pharmacology and Drug Therapy in Nursing, 2nd ed. Philadelphia: J. B. Lippincott Co., 1979.

# NURSING CARE
# DURING CHILDBEARING

Directions: Read each study question carefully. Select one answer from the four choices presented that you think answers the question correctly. There is only one correct answer to each question. Use the answer key to find out whether the answer you selected is the correct one. Read carefully the explanations for the patient situations presented in the study questions, paying particular attention to the explanations for any questions you missed.

Mrs. Mary Lyons, 32 years old and a multigravida, is in the 35th week of her pregnancy. She is admitted to the hospital in active labor.

---

1. Mrs. Lyons is expected to deliver a premature infant. Which of these aspects of Mrs. Lyons's care requires judicious consideration?

   A. The use of narcotics for Mrs. Lyons.

   B. The method used to determine the duration of Mrs. Lyons's contractions.

   C. The techniques used in cleansing Mrs. Lyons's perineum.

   D. The position Mrs. Lyons is asked to assume.

2. Mrs. Lyons is now in the transitional phase of labor, and she has a need for all of the following measures. The nurse should give priority to which of these measures?

   A. Providing a quiet environment for her.

   B. Having a supporting person with her.

   C. Giving her an explanation of the progress of her labor.

   D. Keeping the area under her buttocks clean and dry.

3. Mrs. Lyons's membranes rupture at the end of the first stage of labor. The nurse should check fetal heart tones immediately for which of these purposes?

   A. To determine if premature separation of the placenta has occurred.

   B. To detect evidence of possible compression of the cord.

   C. To evaluate the force exerted on the cervix.

   D. To assess the pressure in the umbilical vessels.

Mrs. Lyons delivers a boy weighing 4 lb. 11 oz. (2,126 gm.). She is planning to breast-feed her baby. The nurse performs the initial newborn assessment.

---

4. The ABSENCE of which of these reflexes in Baby Boy Lyons would be most indicative of neurologic damage?

   A. Moro.

   B. Tonic neck.

   C. Babinski.

   D. Grasp.

5. Six hours after the delivery, the nurse observes that Mrs. Lyons's uterine fundus is firm, 2 fingerbreadths above the umbilicus, and palpable in the right side of her abdomen. Mrs. Lyons also has a heavy flow of lochia rubra.

   The nurse should take which of these actions first?

   A. Palpate Mrs. Lyons's bladder.

   B. Take Mrs. Lyons's vital signs.

   C. Massage Mrs. Lyons's uterus vigorously.

   D. Place an ice bag on Mrs. Lyons's fundus.

6. Since Mrs. Lyons is to breast-feed her baby, the nurse gives her all of the following instructions. Which one is for the purpose of minimizing soreness of the nipples?

   A. "Wear a supportive brassiere."

   B. "Express a little milk manually before nursing."

   C. "Increase nursing time gradually."

   D. "Assume a comfortable position when nursing."

7. On the third postpartum day, Mrs. Lyons complains about soreness and fullness in her breasts and says that she does not want to breast-feed her infant until her breasts are less sore.

The nurse should take which of these actions?

A. Suggest that Mrs. Lyons restrict fluids to temporarily suppress lactation and to reduce engorgement of her breasts.

B. Tell Mrs. Lyons that her breast engorgement is a contraindication for breast-feeding, and that the baby should be started on formula feedings.

C. Show Mrs. Lyons how to apply a breast binder to relieve discomfort and to decrease the production of milk.

D. Explain to Mrs. Lyons that the infant's sucking will promote the flow of milk and reduce breast discomfort.

---------------------------------------------
Mrs. Lyons is discharged. When Baby Boy Lyons has gained sufficient weight, plans are made for his discharge.
---------------------------------------------

8. Since Baby Boy Lyons was born prematurely, the nurse should give Mrs. Lyons which of these instructions about his care?

A. "Keep him isolated from other family members for several weeks."

B. "Care for him as for any normal newborn infant."

C. "Provide humidity in his environment."

D. "Plan to stimulate him periodically both physically and emotionally."

---------------------------------------------
When Mrs. Lyons is 6 weeks postpartum, she has a checkup in the clinic. Her husband accompanies her.
---------------------------------------------

9. The Lyonses ask the nurse for information about family planning. The nurse's response should be influenced most by which of these considerations?

A. The health of the mother.

B. The age of the couple.

C. The nurse's own philosophy on contraception.

D. The expressed request of the couple.

10. Mrs. Lyons asks how the hormones in oral contraceptives prevent pregnancy. The nurse should explain that the chief effect of the estrogen in oral contraceptives is to

A. release the luteinizing hormone.

B. control peristalsis in the fallopian tubes.

C. suppress follicular growth.

D. stimulate gonadotropic function.

---------------------------------------------
Mrs. Ann Clark, 21 years old, is two months pregnant when she attends the antepartal clinic for the first time. This is her first pregnancy.
---------------------------------------------

11. During Mrs. Clark's first visit to the antepartal clinic, she should have which of these routine procedures?

A. Amniography.

B. Papanicolaou smear.

C. Ultrasonic scanning of the abdomen.

D. Fasting blood sugar determination.

12. Mrs. Clark should be instructed that it will be essential to contact the clinic if she develops which of these symptoms?

A. Recurrent heartburn.

B. Difficulty in sleeping.

C. Persistent headache.

D. Urinary frequency.

---

Mrs. Clark's pregnancy progresses normally. At term, when she comes to the hospital in early active labor, her membranes are intact.

---

13. Which of these occurrences would indicate that Mrs. Clark is approaching the end of the first stage of labor?

A. Her contractions decrease in strength.

B. Her membranes rupture spontaneously.

C. She complains of a backache.

D. She says she has a desire to move her bowels.

14. At which of these times would it be appropriate to encourage Mrs. Clark to bear down with her contractions?

A. After the membranes have ruptured.

B. After her cervix is fully dilated.

C. After she expresses the desire to push with a contraction.

D. After she is having contractions every 2 to 3 minutes.

---

Mrs. Clark delivers a 7-lb., 8-oz. (3,402-gm.) boy over an episiotomy. Mrs. Clark is transferred to the postpartum unit and Baby Boy Clark is transferred to the nursery.

---

15. On Mrs. Clark's second postpartum day, she says that she has been urinating very often and in large amounts. Mrs. Clark should be given which of these explanations of diuresis during the early postpartum period?

A. The bladder has become relaxed.

B. The uterus is exerting pressure on the bladder.

C. Excess body fluid accumulated during pregnancy is being excreted.

D. A low-grade infection may be present.

16. Mrs. Clark asks the nurse how long her lochial flow will last. The nurse should explain that lochial discharge usually lasts for approximately

A. 5 days.

B. 9 days.

C. 4 weeks.

D. 6 weeks.

Mrs. Debra Lang, a 32-year-old primigravida, is at term when she is admitted to the labor room in early active labor. Her membranes are intact, and she is having contractions lasting 30 to 45 seconds every 6 to 8 minutes.

Mrs. Lang's antepartum record indicates an obstetrical conjugate of 9.5 cm. and a possible borderline cephalopelvic disproportion. Mrs. Lang is to have a period of trial labor to evaluate the possibility of a vaginal delivery.

17. Mrs. Lang's record includes all of the following data. Which information indicates that Mrs. Lang's labor and delivery are UNLIKELY to follow a normal course?

    A. The mucus plug is intact.

    B. The fetal weight is approximately 6 1/2 lb. (2,948 gm.).

    C. The cervix is dilated 3 cm.

    D. The fetus is in vertex presentation with the head unengaged.

18. During labor, Mrs. Lang has an episode of pallor, sweating, and tachycardia. Because the nurse suspects supine hypotensive syndrome, which of these measures should be taken?

    A. Positioning Mrs. Lang on her side.

    B. Placing Mrs. Lang flat in bed.

    C. Elevating Mrs. Lang's legs.

    D. Giving Mrs. Lang a few inhalations of oxygen.

After an unsuccessful period of trial labor, Mrs. Lang has a cesarean section. She is delivered of a 7-lb. (3,175-gm.) boy.

19. Since Baby Boy Lang was delivered by cesarean section, a finding that he would NOT have that occurs in infants delivered vaginally is

    A. breast engorgement.

    B. caput succedaneum.

    C. transient tachypnea.

    D. open posterior fontanel.

Mrs. Lang is transferred to the postpartum unit and Baby Boy Lang is transferred to the newborn nursery.

20. During the early postpartum period, which of these measures will be more important for Mrs. Lang than for a woman who delivered vaginally?

    A. Giving perineal care.

    B. Encouraging deep-breathing exercises.

    C. Observing for an elevated temperature.

    D. Providing for periods of rest.

---
There has been a severe storm. At 2 a.m., Mr. Ned Samson telephones his neighbor, who is a nurse, and says, "My wife's labor has started. She's ten days early. I know I can't get her to the hospital." The nurse responds to Mr. Samson's request for help and goes to the Samson home.

---

21. Mrs. Samson's labor progresses rapidly, and the nurse assesses that she is at the end of the first stage of labor. Mrs. Samson suddenly starts to scream and cry. Which of these approaches should the nurse use?

   A. Explain to Mrs. Samson that she needs to conserve her energy for the next phase of labor.

   B. Ask Mrs. Samson to try her usual methods of relaxation.

   C. Caution Mrs. Samson that she is prolonging her labor.

   D. Perform breathing exercises with Mrs. Samson.


22. The nurse observes that the baby's head is beginning to emerge. At this time, it is essential for the nurse to take which of these actions?

   A. Encourage Mrs. Samson to bear down with contractions.

   B. Reassure Mrs. Samson that her labor is almost over.

   C. Rotate the infant's head.

   D. Prevent rapid expulsion of the infant's head.

---
Mrs. Samson delivers a girl.

---

23. Mr. Samson is present at the delivery. He asks the nurse why the umbilical cord is not cut immediately. The nurse should give him which of these explanations?

   A. "The blood vessels in the cord will collapse spontaneously as the infant's respirations are established."

   B. "The circulation of blood within the cord ceases soon after the baby is born."

   C. "Thromboplastin will be released by the placenta as it separates to clot the blood in the cord."

   D. "A substance is released from the placenta to block circulation to the cord."


24. All of the following measures should be taken after Mrs. Samson delivers the placenta. Which one should have priority?

   A. Maintaining a firm uterine fundus.

   B. Examining the perineum.

   C. Checking Mrs. Samson's pulse rate.

   D. Keeping Mrs. Samson warm.

Mrs. Katherine Leonard, 30 years old, is 10 weeks pregnant. She is attending the antepartal clinic. Mrs. Leonard is Rh negative and her husband is Rh positive. She has a 6-year-old son who is Rh positive. A year ago she had a spontaneous abortion at 5 weeks' gestation. Mrs. Leonard never received anti-D immunoglobulin (RHoGAM).

25. Mrs. Leonard is to take ferrous sulfate tablets. Oral iron preparations may have which of these side effects?

   A. An increase of melanin deposits in the skin.

   B. Gastrointestinal disturbances.

   C. An acceleration of the formation of plaque deposits on the teeth.

   D. A metallic aftertaste.

26. Mrs. Leonard is taught about foods that are high in iron. The teaching will have been effective if Mrs. Leonard selects which of these groups of foods as highest in iron?

   A. Kidney beans, broccoli, and eggs.

   B. Processed cheese, green beans, and rice.

   C. Chicken, carrots, and skim milk.

   D. Tuna fish, celery, and grapefruit.

27. Mrs. Leonard has a hematocrit determination done and the results indicate that her hematocrit is low. This finding is most likely to be due to which of these changes during pregnancy?

   A. Expanding blood volume.

   B. Decreasing absorption of minerals from the gastrointestinal tract.

   C. Hemolysis of red blood cells by Rh antibodies.

   D. A shortened lifespan of red blood cells.

28. Mrs. Leonard has an indirect Coombs' test done at intervals during her pregnancy. The purpose of this test is to

   A. identify fetal red blood cells in maternal blood.

   B. determine the level of anti-D antibodies in maternal serum.

   C. measure the rate of hemolysis of maternal red blood cells.

   D. detect an elevation of maternal bilirubin.

At term, Mrs. Leonard is admitted to the hospital in active labor and delivers a boy who is Rh positive. When Baby Boy Leonard is 24 hours old, he has a positive Coombs' test, and his serum bilirubin is 8 mg. per 100 ml. of blood.

29. Baby Boy Leonard is having phototherapy. In addition to covering his eyes, which of these measures should be included in his care during the treatment?

   A. Lubricating his skin with oil.

   B. Reducing his environmental stimuli.

   C. Monitoring his urine output.

   D. Checking his urine for protein.

Mr. and Mrs. Caron are attending a genetic
counseling center. The Carons have a
3-year-old child who has cystic fibrosis. The
center employs a nurse.

30. Mrs. Caron says to the nurse, "Considering
the risks, we are not sure about having
another child. What do you think we should
do?" Since cystic fibrosis is transmitted
as an autosomal recessive disorder, which
of these statements about the chance of the
Carons' next child having the defect is
accurate?

A. Whether this defect will occur in their
next child depends on the sex of that
child.

B. The defect may affect the third child
but not the second one.

C. There is a 50-50 chance that their next
child will have this defect.

D. The chances are one in four that this
defect will appear in their next child.

---

Mrs. Caron becomes pregnant and attends the
antepartal clinic regularly. At term, she is
admitted to the hospital in labor.

---

31. When Mrs. Caron is admitted to the
obstetric unit, the baseline fetal heart
rate is 128; one hour later, it is 165.
This type of change in fetal heart rate is
most likely to be related to which of these
occurrences?

A. The fetus has a mild hypoxia.

B. The head of the fetus has entered the
true pelvis.

C. The mother's anxiety level has increased.

D. The cervix is fully dilated.

---

Mrs. Caron's labor progresses normally, and she
delivers an apparently normal girl.

---

32. To promote the maternal-infant bonding
process, which of these procedures for the
baby should be withheld until after Mrs.
Caron holds her baby?

A. Taking the baby's footprints.

B. Administering vitamin $K_1$ to the baby.

C. Administering prophylactic eyedrops to
the baby.

D. Suctioning the baby's oral cavity.

---

Mrs. Caron and her baby are transferred to a
rooming-in unit. Mrs. Caron is to breast-feed
her baby.

---

33. Baby Girl Caron awakens 2 1/2 hours after a
feeding. Mrs. Caron attempts to feed her
infant, but the infant does not seem to be
interested in a feeding. The nurse should
give Mrs. Caron which of these suggestions
at this time?

A. "Wait until she starts to get fussy
before trying to feed her."

B. "She may want a diaper change before
being fed."

C. "Perhaps she'll take a little water
first."

D. "Try touching her at the corners of her
mouth."

34. Mrs. Caron says she is having afterpains while breast-feeding her baby. Which of these actions should the nurse include in Mrs. Caron's care about a half hour before Mrs. Caron feeds her baby?

A. Suggest that Mrs. Caron perform relaxation techniques.

B. Encourage Mrs. Caron to void.

C. Administer the prescribed analgesic to Mrs. Caron.

D. Teach Mrs. Caron to massage her uterine fundus.

------------------------------------------------
Mrs. Sally Mann, a 20-year-old primigravida, is receiving antepartal care from a private physician. Mrs. Mann is in the 12th week of her pregnancy. The nurse in the physician's office is discussing antepartal care with Mrs. Mann.
------------------------------------------------

35. Mrs. Mann says to the nurse, "I read that even if you had been eating a balanced diet before becoming pregnant, once you become pregnant, your protein requirement increases. Why is that?"

Which of these explanations by the nurse would give Mrs. Mann correct information?

A. "The end products of maternal protein digestion are stored by the fetus for use in the neonatal period."

B. "The kidneys of a pregnant women tend to excrete protein at a slightly higher rate than those of a nonpregnant woman."

C. "The development of the fetus is dependent on maternal protein intake."

D. "The maternal metabolic rate is increased during pregnancy."

36. In the fifth month of pregnancy, Mrs. Mann should expect which of these effects of pregnancy to occur?

A. Urinary frequency.

B. Difficulty in breathing when in a recumbent position.

C. Tenderness around the umbilicus.

D. Quickening.

37. Mrs. Mann is now in the seventh month of her pregnancy. She says to the nurse, "I understand why drugs cannot be taken in the first months of pregnancy, but why would taking drugs late in the pregnancy also be bad?" The nurse should explain that drugs may have which of these effects throughout pregnancy?

A. Drugs may change the anatomical structure of the placental barrier.

B. Drugs may cause structural deformities in the fetus.

C. Drugs may change biochemical functioning in the fetus.

D. Drugs may be trapped in the placenta when they bind with protein.

------------------------------------------------
At term, Mrs. Mann is admitted to the hospital in labor. Her labor progresses normally until her cervix is 5 cm. dilated, but the cervix does not dilate any further. X-rays are taken, and a cephalopelvic disproportion is diagnosed.
------------------------------------------------

38. To give Mrs. Mann accurate information about her condition, the nurse should explain that a cephalopelvic disproportion exists under which of these conditions?

A. The circumference of the fetal head is larger than its occipitomental diameter.

B. The circumference of the fetal head is too large to fit through the internal os.

C. The occipitofrontal diameter of the fetal head is larger than its bitemporal diameter.

D. The biparietal diameter of the fetal head is too large to pass through the midpelvis.

---------------------------------------------
Mrs. Mann has a cesarean section and is
delivered of a girl weighing 7 lb. 5 oz.
(3,317 gm.).  Baby Girl Mann is transferred to
the nursery.
---------------------------------------------

39. Baby Girl Mann has hyaline membrane
    disease.  Which of these pathologic changes
    occurs with this disease?

    A. The production of surfactant increases.

    B. The bronchi overexpand.

    C. The alveoli tend to collapse.

    D. The lining of the bronchi is irritated
       by a lipoprotein.


---------------------------------------------
Mrs. Laura Cannon, 18 years old, visits the
antepartal clinic.  She is about 10 weeks
pregnant.  This is her first pregnancy.
---------------------------------------------

40. Which of these statements, if made by Mrs.
    Cannon, would reflect a normal
    physiological development of pregnancy?

    A. "I have a little spotting at the time I
       would have my usual menstrual period."

    B. "My bras don't fit anymore."

    C. "I'm sleeping about an hour less than I
       used to."

    D. "I have a white vaginal discharge that
       makes me itch."


41. Mrs. Cannon's nutritional status before
    pregnancy should be assessed because of
    which of these occurrences during the first
    trimester of pregnancy?

    A. Increased urinary output.

    B. Development of fetal organs.

    C. Maternal susceptibility to infection.

    D. Depletion of maternal stores of vitamins
       by the fetus.

42. When Mrs. Cannon is 7 months pregnant, she
    gains 6 lb. (2,722 gm.) in 2 weeks.  To
    take appropriate action, the nurse should
    make which of these interpretations of Mrs.
    Cannon's weight gain?

    A. It is indicative of a poor understanding
       of good nutritional practices.

    B. It is indicative of a problem in a
       teenage primigravida.

    C. It may be due to causes other than an
       excessive caloric intake.

    D. It is expected for this period of
       gestation in young primigravidas.


---------------------------------------------
At term, Mrs. Cannon is admitted to the
hospital, and she delivers a girl.
---------------------------------------------

43. An assessment of Baby Girl Cannon is made.
    Her hands and feet are dusky, dark blue,
    and cool to the touch.  Which of these
    nursing diagnoses should be made?

    A. Interruption in thermoregulation related
       to a minimal amount of body fat.

    B. Interruption in glucose metabolism
       related to an immature liver.

    C. Interruption in oxygenation related to
       fetal hemoglobin.

    D. Interruption in hemodynamics related to
       vasomotor instability.

44. Baby Girl Cannon develops hyper-bilirubinemia and is to have phototherapy. The physician discusses this situation with Mrs. Cannon. After the physician leaves, Mrs. Cannon is obviously upset. To meet Mrs. Cannon's needs at this time, the nurse should take which of these actions?

A. Inform Mrs. Cannon that the baby's growth and development will proceed normally following the planned phototherapy.

B. Tell Mrs. Cannon that the procedure is a safe one and that the baby will be cured.

C. Let Mrs. Cannon know that the nurse is interested in her and is willing to listen if she wishes to talk.

D. Explain to Mrs. Cannon what phototherapy is and how it is done.

45. On her third day postpartum, Mrs. Cannon becomes withdrawn and teary. The nurse should take which of these approaches?

A. Provide privacy for Mrs. Cannon and tell her that her feelings will be discussed with the physician.

B. Ask Mrs. Cannon if there is anything she would like the nurse to do and whether she would like to see her baby.

C. Explain to Mrs. Cannon that her feelings are not unusual and institute measures that will indicate interest in her.

D. Encourage Mrs. Cannon to focus on the joys of motherhood and plan activities with her that will be diverting.

---------------------------------------------------
Mrs. Lila Bertram, a 23-year-old typist, visits the antepartal clinic for the first time. She has a pregnancy of about 10 weeks' gestation. This is her first pregnancy.
---------------------------------------------------

46. At 10 weeks' gestation, Mrs. Bertram should have which of these signs of pregnancy?

A. Urinary frequency.

B. Enlargement of the abdomen.

C. Lightening.

D. Quickening.

47. Mrs. Bertram says, "I'm not as happy as I thought I'd be about being pregnant. My husband and I want a family, but we had hoped to have more money saved." The nurse should make which of these responses initially?

A. "You seem to have mixed feelings about being pregnant."

B. "Your pregnancy has upset you."

C. "You will be happier about your pregnancy after you have talked with your husband."

D. "Your pregnancy will not interfere with your plans for several months."

48. Mrs. Bertram asks the nurse about taking nonprescription drugs for a headache or for symptoms of a cold. Which of these responses would give Mrs. Bertram correct information?

A. "The drugs that you can obtain without a prescription are not harmful."

B. "Drugs taken in the first trimester of pregnancy may be harmful to the fetus."

C. "You should limit the use of drugs to those required to relieve specific symptoms of pregnancy."

D. "Drugs would harm the fetus only if they have a harmful effect on the mother."

49. Since Mrs. Bertram works as a typist, it would be most important for her to follow which of these practices?

A. Walking around periodically.

B. Using a chair that allows her to stretch backward.

C. Sitting on a soft cushion.

D. Taking deep breaths at regular intervals.

---

Mrs. Bertram's pregnancy progresses normally. She is admitted to the hospital at term in early active labor.

---

50. Shortly after admission, Mrs. Bertram's membranes rupture spontaneously. The nurse should take which of these actions first?

A. Time the uterine contractions.

B. Assess the fetal heart tones.

C. Count Mrs. Bertram's pulse.

D. Take Mrs. Bertram's blood pressure.

51. When Mrs. Bertram is in the second stage of labor, which of these actions is it most important for the nurse to take?

A. Encourage her to empty her bladder frequently.

B. Provide her with extra warmth.

C. Place her in a lithotomy position.

D. Remain with her.

---

Mrs. Bertram delivers a 6-lb. (2,722-gm.) girl spontaneously. Mrs. Bertram is transferred to the postpartum unit and Baby Girl Bertram is transferred to the nursery. Baby Girl Bertram is to be bottle-fed.

---

52. When Baby Girl Bertram is bottle-fed for the first time, she will most probably receive which of these solutions?

A. Sterile water.

B. Dilute formula.

C. Normal saline.

D. Twenty-percent glucose.

53. When helping Mrs. Bertram to bottle-feed her baby for the first time, the nurse should give her which of these instructions?

A. "Don't allow any air bubbles to collect in the baby's bottle."

B. "Encourage the baby to suck by rubbing the area under her chin."

C. "Shake the nipple in the baby's mouth if she stops sucking."

D. "Hold the baby so that she is in close contact with your body."

54. When Baby Girl Bertram's mattress is struck sharply, her arms fly up and out and her legs draw up. This response is characteristic of which of these reflexes?

A. Babinski.

B. Tonic neck.

C. Moro.

D. Parachute.

---
Mrs. Fay Lubek, a 27-year-old multigravida, is admitted to the hospital in active labor. She has had an uneventful pregnancy. She delivers a girl weighing 7 lb. 8 oz. (3,402 gm.) over an episiotomy. Mrs. Lubek is transferred to the postpartum unit and Baby Girl Lubek is transferred to the nursery. Mrs. Lubek plans to breast-feed her baby. She bottle-fed her first baby.
---

55. The nurse's assessment of Baby Girl Lubek reveals a white mucous discharge from the infant's vagina. The nurse should take which of these actions first?

   A. Keep the infant's perineal area exposed to the air.

   B. Check the infant's temperature.

   C. Describe the finding on the infant's chart.

   D. Consult the mother's chart to see what medications were administered to her during labor.

56. In comparison with a primipara, a multipara such as Mrs. Lubek is more likely to have which of these problems?

   A. Afterpains.

   B. Cystitis.

   C. Breast engorgement.

   D. Postpartum psychosis.

57. Mrs. Lubek tells the nurse that her husband does not believe in breast-feeding. Which of these comments should the nurse make?

   A. "How long do you plan to breast-feed your baby?"

   B. "Do you know what your husband's objections to breast-feeding are?"

   C. "Maybe you should give the baby a bottle instead."

   D. "As you and the baby do well at home, your husband will probably change his mind."

58. Twelve hours after delivery, Mrs. Lubek's uterine fundus is one and one half fingerbreadths above the umbilicus, displaced slightly to the right, and firm.

   These findings are most probably indicative of

   A. subvolution.

   B. normal involution.

   C. bladder distention.

   D. retention of lochia.

59. On the second postpartum day, Mrs. Lubek says to the nurse, "I've had to change my sanitary napkins very often this morning. They get soaked with bright red blood." Which of these actions should the nurse take first?

   A. Advise Mrs. Lubek to stay in bed.

   B. Notify Mrs. Lubek's physician.

   C. Take Mrs. Lubek's vital signs.

   D. Check Mrs. Lubek's uterine fundus.

60. When Mrs. Lubek is being taught about breast care, which of these instructions should be included?

   A. "To prevent sore nipples, keep a moist compress over the nipples between feedings."

   B. "To prevent sore nipples, be sure the baby has the whole nipple and most of the areola in her mouth during feedings."

   C. "To prevent a breast infection, wash the nipples with soap and water before each feeding."

   D. "To prevent a breast infection, give the baby a small amount of sterile water before each feeding."

---
Mrs. Toni Vinton, 32 years old, has a
4-year-old child. Mrs. Vinton comes to the
antepartal clinic when she is two months
pregnant. She has had diabetes mellitus for
three years. Her diabetic condition has been
controlled by diet and insulin. Four weeks
before the expected date of delivery, Mrs.
Vinton is admitted to the hospital to have an
amniocentesis.
---

61. Mrs. Vinton is having an amniocentesis
    performed near term for which of these
    purposes?

    A. To remove excess amniotic fluid.

    B. To assess the maturity of the fetus.

    C. To measure the pressure of the amniotic
       fluid.

    D. To obtain a blood specimen from the
       fetus.

62. Since Mrs. Vinton has diabetes mellitus,
    she may be delivered before term by
    cesarean section to prevent

    A. the development of diabetes in the fetus.

    B. alterations in her insulin requirements.

    C. tearing of her perineum.

    D. fetal death.

---
Mrs. Vinton is admitted to the labor and
delivery unit two weeks before her expected
date of delivery. Mrs. Vinton is not in active
labor.
---

63. Mrs. Vinton's labor is induced. She is
    receiving oxytocin injection (Pitocin)
    intravenously. Which of these signs would
    be indicative of an UNTOWARD effect of this
    medication?

    A. Fetal heart rate of 155 beats per minute.

    B. Appearance of bloody show.

    C. Uterine contractions lasting more than
       90 seconds.

    D. Radial pulse rate of 92 beats per minute.

64. Because Mrs. Vinton has received an
    oxytocic drug, it will be necessary to
    include which of these measures in her care?

    A. Monitoring her blood pressure.

    B. Administering oxygen by cannula at 2
       liters a minute.

    C. Maintaining her in a side-lying position.

    D. Testing her urine for the presence of
       protein.

65. Mrs. Vinton's membranes rupture. The nurse
    should take which of these actions first?

    A. Check the fetal heart rate.

    B. Examine Mrs. Vinton's perineum.

    C. Change Mrs. Vinton's perineal pad.

    D. Encourage Mrs. Vinton to pant with each
       contraction.

---
Mrs. Anna Little, age 26, attends the
antepartal clinic for the first time. She is
10 weeks pregnant. This is Mrs. Little's first
pregnancy.
---

66. Mrs. Little says to the nurse, "I've always
    wanted to have a baby. I thought I'd be
    happy, but now I'm having second
    thoughts." Which of these responses should
    the nurse make initially?

    A. "You'll feel different once you feel the
       baby move."

    B. "Tell me how your husband feels about
       your being pregnant."

    C. "You have mixed feelings about being
       pregnant now."

    D. "Motherly feelings sometimes take a long
       time to develop."

67. The nurse is reviewing Mrs. Little's nutritional needs with her. The following foods are typical of those that Mrs. Little eats for lunch. Which of these menus is highest in protein?

A. Bacon, lettuce, and tomato sandwich and an apple.

B. Peanut butter sandwich and lemon pudding.

C. Jelly sandwich and a banana.

D. Cream cheese and olive sandwich and flavored gelatin.

---

Mrs. Little is now in the seventh month of her pregnancy. The Littles plan to attend preparation-for-childbirth classes that use the psychoprophylactic (Lamaze) method, and Mrs. Little has decided that she will breast-feed her baby.

---

68. To prepare Mrs. Little's nipples for breast-feeding, she should be given which of these instructions?

A. "Do not handle your nipples unnecessarily."

B. "Apply alcohol to your nipples twice a day."

C. "Wear a brassiere that fits loosely over your nipples."

D. "Rub your nipples gently with a towel every day."

69. Mrs. Little is talking with the nurse about her plans for her infant. Mrs. Little says, "It's bad luck to buy things for a baby before it's born. The more you buy, the greater the possibility that the baby will be sick."

Which of these responses by the nurse would be best?

A. "You are entitled to your belief. Besides, a newborn baby doesn't need very much."

B. "I can understand why you wouldn't want to accumulate baby things while you are pregnant. If anything happened to the baby, they would be a reminder."

C. "Please explain how buying a few things can possibly affect the health of your baby."

D. "The time at which you buy things for the baby is up to you. However, there are no indications that your baby will be anything but healthy."

70. In the eighth month of her pregnancy, Mrs. Little experiences a short episode of painless bright red vaginal bleeding. Mrs. Little is to have a 24-hour specimen of urine collected for estriol level determinations. The purpose of this test is to assess

A. the response of the adrenal glands to stress.

B. the effect of blood loss on the kidneys.

C. the age of the fetus.

D. the functioning of the placenta.

71. Mrs. Little's pregnancy progresses normally. She should be instructed to come to the hospital immediately if which of these events occurs?

    A. She has a sudden gush of clear fluid from her vagina.

    B. She has persistent back pain.

    C. She has contractions for a period of 3 hours.

    D. She has an episode of nausea and vomiting.

---
At term, Mrs. Little is admitted to the hospital in labor. Mr. Little is with her.
---

72. When Mrs. Little is admitted, it is most important to ask her which of these questions?

    A. "When did you eat last?"

    B. "Have you had a bowel movement within the last twenty-four hours?"

    C. "Have you been urinating at least every two hours?"

    D. "When was your last antepartal visit?"

73. Mrs. Little nears the end of the first stage of labor. When Mrs. Little is having a contraction, the nurse should take which of these actions?

    A. Provide a soft object for her to squeeze.

    B. Do the related breathing exercises with her.

    C. Help her to remain in a lithotomy position.

    D. Have her gently apply downward pressure on her uterine fundus.

74. When Mrs. Little's cervix is fully dilated, she asks the nurse for some medication for pain. The nurse's response should be based on which of these understandings about the effects of pain medication given at this time?

    A. It may interfere with the woman's ability to bond with her infant.

    B. It may lower blood pressure to a hazardous level.

    C. It may cause a precipitous delivery.

    D. It may affect the infant's ability to adapt to extrauterine life.

---
Mrs. Little has an episiotomy and delivers a girl.
---

75. Baby Girl Little's 1-minute Apgar score is 8. Which of these assessments is included in the procedure for obtaining an Apgar score?

    A. Blood pressure.

    B. Gestational age.

    C. Response of reflexes.

    D. Presence of congenital defects.

76. Shortly after delivery, Mrs. Little receives a dose of methylergonovine (Methergine) maleate. Methergine is given during the postpartum period for which of these purposes?

    A. To promote urinary output.

    B. To minimize breast engorgement.

    C. To increase blood pressure.

    D. To control uterine bleeding.

77. Silver nitrate drops are instilled into Baby Girl Little's eyes to prevent

A. retrolental fibroplasia.

B. ophthalmia neonatorum.

C. syphilis iritis.

D. chemical conjunctivitis.

---

Mrs. Little is transferred to the postpartum unit and Baby Girl Little is transferred to the nursery.

---

78. When Baby Girl Little is being admitted to the nursery, it is important to take which of these actions first?

A. Weigh her.

B. Measure her head and chest circumferences.

C. Provide her with warmth.

D. Apply an antiseptic to her cord.

79. Shortly after Baby Girl Little is born, Mr. Little says, "I hope I can learn to enjoy her. I really was expecting a boy." Which of these measures is likely to facilitate bonding between Mr. Little and his baby?

A. Encouraging him to discuss his feelings with his wife.

B. Giving him opportunity to take care of the baby.

C. Pointing out to him the positive aspects of having a healthy baby.

D. Explaining to him how important affection is in the emotional development of a baby.

80. During the first 24 hours of life, which of these findings, if present in Baby Girl Little, would be indicative of an abnormality?

A. A yellowish tinge of the sclerae.

B. White spots on the sides of the nose.

C. The skin over the torso is mottled.

D. The palms and soles have a bluish color.

81. Mrs. Little and the nurse discuss rooming-in. The basic purpose of rooming-in would best be explained by which of these statements?

A. "Parents who learn how to care for their baby in the hospital are not anxious when they take the baby home."

B. "In rooming-in, babies are more content and cry less."

C. "Knowing the needs of a newborn helps mothers to schedule household activities more efficiently."

D. "Parents who have their babies with them more quickly develop the feeling that they and their baby are a family."

82. On the afternoon of the third postpartum day, Mrs. Little is crying. Which of these actions should the nurse take first?

A. Offer to stay with her.

B. Allow her privacy.

C. Encourage her to ambulate.

D. Check to see if she has an order for a sedative.

83. Mrs. Simpson is to have a pelvic
    examination.  She says to the nurse, "I
    know this is ridiculous, but I hate being
    examined."  To give Mrs. Simpson support
    during the examination, the nurse should
    take which of these actions?

    A. Instruct Mrs. Simpson to alternately
       relax and contract her perineal muscles.

    B. Encourage Mrs. Simpson to take slow,
       deep breaths through her mouth.

    C. Tell Mrs. Simpson that the nurse will
       hold her hands.

    D. Remind Mrs. Simpson frequently to relax.


84. The nurse is reviewing Mrs. Simpson's
    nutritional needs with her.  Mrs. Simpson
    says that she usually has only coffee and
    toast for breakfast.  Which of these foods,
    if added to her breakfast, would provide
    the most iron?

    A. A medium banana.

    B. A bowl of oatmeal.

    C. A serving of bacon.

    D. A cup of milk.


----------------------------------------
Mrs. Simpson has an uneventful pregnancy.  At
term, she is admitted to the hospital in active
labor.
----------------------------------------

85. Mrs. Simpson has an epidural type of
    anesthesia.  After Mrs. Simpson receives
    the anesthesia, the nurse should take which
    of these actions first?

    A. Take her blood pressure.

    B. Check her pedal pulses.

    C. Place her in lithotomy position.

    D. Time her contractions.


----------------------------------------
Mrs. Simpson's labor progresses normally, and
she delivers a boy.
----------------------------------------

86. One-half hour after delivery, Mrs.
    Simpson's uterine fundus is firm and two
    fingerbreadths below the umbilicus, and her
    lochia is bright red.  She complains of
    feeling slightly chilly and thirsty.  These
    findings are indicative of

    A. subinvolution.

    B. bladder distention.

    C. normal postpartal adjustment.

    D. impending shock.


----------------------------------------
Mrs. Simpson is transferred to the postpartum
unit and Baby Boy Simpson is transferred to the
nursery.
----------------------------------------

87. One hour after birth, Baby Boy Simpson's
    respirations are 70 per minute, and he has
    some sternal retraction.  In addition to
    assessing the baby's need for suctioning,
    the nurse should take which of these
    actions?

    A. Keep the infant warm.

    B. Place the infant in a head-dependent
       position.

    C. Check the infant's Moro reflex.

    D. Palpate the infant's abdomen.


88. Baby Boy Simpson's blood is drawn to make
    blood gas determinations.  The results are:
    pH., 7.20; pO$_2$, 40 mm. Hg.; pCO$_2$, 70
    mm. Hg.  Based on this data, which of these
    medications should be available for
    administration to the infant?

    A. Calcium gluconate.

    B. Nalorphine hydrochloride (Nalline).

    C. Epinephrine hydrochloride (Adrenalin).

    D. Sodium bicarbonate.

89. To evaluate the progress of Mrs. Simpson's uterine involution, the nurse should periodically make which of these assessments?

A. The volume of each of Mrs. Simpson's voidings.

B. The tone of Mrs. Simpson's abdominal muscles.

C. The appearance of Mrs. Simpson's perineum.

D. The character of Mrs. Simpson's lochia.

90. Baby Boy Simpson develops thrush during the first few days of life. The primary source of thrush is usually

A. the hands of personnel.

B. formula equipment.

C. bassinet linen.

D. the mother's birth canal.

---

Mrs. Elaine Roth, 27 years old, is in the 30th week of her second pregnancy. She is receiving care at the antepartal clinic.

---

91. Mrs. Roth calls the clinic because she has some vaginal spotting. To assess Mrs. Roth's situation, it is essential for the nurse to ask which of these questions?

A. "Did you engage in any strenuous physical activity recently?"

B. "Is this around the time of the month that you would normally ovulate?"

C. "Do you have any abdominal pain?"

D. "Did you have this type of bleeding during your first pregnancy?"

---

Mrs. Roth is admitted to the hospital. A diagnosis of placenta previa is made.

---

92. Upon admission, Mrs. Roth is put to bed. While awaiting the arrival of the physician, the nurse should take which of these additional actions?

A. Withhold food and fluids.

B. Massage the uterine fundus.

C. Check Mrs. Roth's urine for the presence of acetone.

D. Place Mrs. Roth in lithotomy position.

---

Mrs. Roth is to remain on bed rest. Three days after admission, Mrs. Roth has frank bleeding, and a 3-lb., 5-oz. (1,503-gm.) boy is delivered by cesarean section. Baby Boy Roth is taken to the premature nursery.

---

93. Because Baby Boy Roth is a premature infant, which of these findings is he likely to have that full-term infants do not have?

A. A chest circumference that is larger than the circumference of his head.

B. Blood vessels that are easily seen through the skin.

C. Breast areolae that are raised.

D. Creases in his soles that extend to his heels.

94. To accurately determine Baby Boy Roth's respiratory rate, the nurse should take which of these actions?

A. Count it before feeding him.

B. Count it while he is at rest.

C. Count it immediately after taking his apical pulse.

D. Count it while he is positioned with his head slightly dependent.

95. To help Mrs. Roth deal with the reality of the situation before Baby Boy Roth is transferred, which of these actions should the nurse take?

A. Inform Mrs. Roth of the neonatal center's visiting hours.

B. Reassure Mrs. Roth that the neonatal center is better equipped to care for the infant.

C. Discuss with Mrs. Roth the type of care the infant will receive.

D. Provide Mrs. Roth with an opportunity to touch the infant.

---
The remainder of the questions are individual questions.
---

96. A woman who is 16 weeks pregnant has an amniocentesis. After the procedure is done, which of these instructions should be given to her?

A. "Stay in bed for eight hours."

B. "Wear a sanitary pad to absorb the drainage."

C. "Notify us if you have any contractions."

D. "Increase your clear fluid intake for the next twenty-four hours."

97. During a visit to the antepartal clinic, a patient who is 30 weeks pregnant complains of leg cramps. The patient's complaint may be related to which of these problems?

A. A phosphorus-calcium imbalance.

B. A decrease in intracellular potassium.

C. Uterine pressure on the pudendal plexus.

D. Insufficient muscle-relaxant hormones.

98. The admission bath for a newborn should be delayed if which of these findings is present in the infant?

A. A cephalohematoma.

B. Acrocyanosis.

C. Milia.

D. Temperature of 96.8°F. (36.0°C.) rectally.

99. When a woman's pregnancy has extended beyond term, it is most important that the nurse should be alert for symptoms of which of these conditions?

A. Placental insufficiency.

B. Prolapse of the umbilical cord.

C. Pregnancy-induced hypertension.

D. Polyhydramnios.

100. A neonate's umbilical cord contains one artery and one vein. Because of this finding, the nurse caring for the neonate should take which of these actions?

A. Assess the infant for evidence of congenital anomalies.

B. Stimulate the infant to cry periodically to increase the depth of respirations.

C. Keep the umbilical stump moist to allow for frequent sampling of blood.

D. Check the infant for evidence of petechiae.

This is the end of the study questions for Nursing Care During Childbearing. Check to see whether you selected the correct answer to each question by using the answer key on page 93. Explanations for the correct answers in each patient situation begin on page 94. Read the explanations carefully, paying particular attention to the explanations for any questions you answered incorrectly. Then select a reference book from the list of recommended texts on page 106. Read the section that pertains to each patient situation presented in the study questions.

# Answer Key to Study Questions
## for Nursing Care During Childbearing

| | | | | |
|---|---|---|---|---|
| 1. A | 21. D | 41. B | 61. B | 81. D |
| 2. B | 22. D | 42. C | 62. D | 82. A |
| 3. B | 23. B | 43. D | 63. C | 83. B |
| 4. A | 24. A | 44. C | 64. A | 84. B |
| 5. A | 25. B | 45. C | 65. A | 85. A |
| 6. C | 26. A | 46. A | 66. C | 86. C |
| 7. D | 27. A | 47. A | 67. B | 87. A |
| 8. B | 28. B | 48. B | 68. D | 88. D |
| 9. D | 29. C | 49. A | 69. D | 89. D |
| 10. C | 30. D | 50. B | 70. D | 90. D |
| 11. B | 31. A | 51. D | 71. A | 91. C |
| 12. C | 32. C | 52. A | 72. A | 92. A |
| 13. D | 33. A | 53. D | 73. B | 93. B |
| 14. B | 34. C | 54. C | 74. D | 94. B |
| 15. C | 35. C | 55. C | 75. C | 95. D |
| 16. C | 36. D | 56. A | 76. D | 96. C |
| 17. D | 37. C | 57. B | 77. B | 97. A |
| 18. A | 38. D | 58. C | 78. C | 98. D |
| 19. B | 39. C | 59. D | 79. B | 99. A |
| 20. B | 40. B | 60. B | 80. A | 100. B |

# Explanations for Study Questions
# for Nursing Care During Childbearing

QUESTIONS 1-10

The onset of labor before term may be caused by fetal, placental, or maternal factors. The use of narcotics causes respiratory depression in the fetus. It is important to know the effect of drugs used during labor on the woman and the fetus.

During the transitional phase of labor, the woman begins to tire and exhibits restlessness and irritability. There is fear of being left alone and a sense of being out of control. Remaining with the woman at this time to provide support is most important.

Following the rupture of the membranes, either spontaneously or due to amniotomy, it is important to determine the possible presence of a prolapsed cord, especially when the pelvic inlet may not be occluded by the fetus.

The initial assessment of preterm infants is most important. The characteristics of preterm infants predispose them to respiratory problems and heat loss. The postnatal period is a time of risk to the continued development of the central nervous system. After assessing the infant at rest, a complete physical assessment is required. The neurological eval-uation should be performed when the infant's status is stable. The absence of the Moro reflex is most indicative of brain damage. Abnormal palmar grasp and absence of the Babinski reflex may indicate a defect in the lower spinal column. The tonic neck reflex may not be present in a preterm infant.

In the early postpartum period, attention should be paid to the possibility of bladder distention, which causes displacement of the uterus and may lead to hemorrhage. Knowledge of normal physical changes in the early postpartum period is basic to performing an accurate assessment of the patient.

Mothers should be informed of problems that may arise when breast-feeding. Initially, breast soreness may occur for about three minutes until the let-down reflex is estab-lished. The breasts should be alternated for feedings and the length of the feeding gradually increased. This will help to establish a milk supply and reduce trauma to the nipples.

When a healthy preterm infant is ready for discharge, the infant will have normal growth and developmental needs.

The approach to family planning should accept the involved couple as responsible for actions taken. The nurse should provide information to the couple so that they can make informed decisions. The hormones used in oral contraceptives achieve their effect by inhibiting ovulation and maintaining a mucus in the cervix that prohibits the entry of sperm. The various methods of family planning as well as the advantages and disadvantages of each should be reviewed.

QUESTIONS 11-16

The first visit for antepartal care is the opportunity to obtain the woman's social and health history. The results of a physical assessment will have implications for the woman and the fetus. In addition to the physical assessment and routine laboratory tests, a Papanicolaou test is done. Fasting blood sugar may be done when the initial urine specimen reveals glycosuria.

Patients should be instructed in all aspects of health care. It is important that they understand the need to report danger signs immediately. These signs include persistent, severe headaches, which may be caused by hypertension.

Knowledge of the expected behavior during the stages of labor will assist in identifying the progress of and response to labor. When the cervix is completely dilated and effaced, the abdominal muscles contract to assist with the expulsion of the fetus. The woman begins to feel the urge to push, which is similar to the urge to defecate. Women should be encouraged to push only after the urge to push occurs with each contraction. The complaint of backache and low abdominal discomfort begins early in labor. Membranes may rupture before labor begins, when the presenting part is not yet engaged, or during the first stage of labor. An amniotomy may be performed as a means of inducing labor or after labor has begun in order to shorten the period of labor.

About 12 to 24 hours after delivery, the urinary output increases due to the need to excrete the 2,000 to 3,000 milliliters of extracellular fluid that is expected in a normal pregnancy. Careful monitoring of urinary output is important.

The assessment of lochia may determine the presence of hemorrhage. The normal changes in lochia serve to indicate the involutional progress of the uterus. The change from lochia rubra to lochia serosa to the cessation of lochia alba takes approximately 4 weeks.

## QUESTIONS 17-20

A variety of fetal positions preclude an uncomplicated vaginal delivery and therefore necessitate cesarean delivery.

The effects of supine hypotension include a decrease in venous return from the lower extremities that compromises the cardiovascular system. A side-lying position will relieve pressure on the vena cava and promote venous blood flow.

Caput succedaneum is a collection of fluid under the infant's scalp that results from sustained pressure by the infant's head on the cervix during labor. Infants delivered by cesarean section are not subject to this trauma.

The nursing management of a woman following a cesarean section requires postoperative measures as well as postpartal measures. Deep-breathing exercises will promote reexpansion of the lungs and prevent pulmonary complications.

## QUESTIONS 21-24

When the active phase of labor begins, there is an intensification of contractions and resulting discomfort. As the woman begins to feel loss of control, constant attendance is supportive. The woman should be encouraged to perform breathing exercises to maintain a breathing pattern. This serves to provide a focus of concentration that will reduce the perception of pain. As the infant's head emerges, it should be supported and delivered slowly to prevent trauma to the head and to the soft tissues of the woman's perineum.

As soon as the infant is delivered, the infant's nose and mouth should be cleared of secretions to promote unobstructed respiration. The delay in clamping and cutting the cord transfers a negligible amount of blood to or from the infant, depending on whether the newborn is held above or below the introitus. The infant's hemoglobin and hematocrit will be higher with a placental infusion of blood.

After the placenta is delivered, it should be carefully examined to make sure that it is intact. The uterine fundus should be palpated at frequent intervals to insure that it remains firm. Loss of uterine tone will result in excessive blood loss.

Rh incompatibility occurs between a woman who is Rh-negative and a fetus that is Rh-positive. RHoGam may be administered to reduce the Rh-antibody titer in an Rh-negative woman after sensitization from an Rh-positive pregnancy. When maternal antibodies cross the placental barrier and attach themselves to the erythrocytes in the fetus, the result is destruction of erythrocytes.

Indirect Coombs' tests on maternal blood monitor the level of anti-D antibodies. Amniocentesis may also be performed to determine the level of bilirubin pigments in amniotic fluid. Elevated bilirubin levels in the newborn result in jaundice within 24 hours and can cause cerebral damage. Special care during treatment of the infant with phototherapy includes preventing dehydration by encouraging fluids between feedings, weighing daily, and monitoring urine output.

The physiological changes in the cardiovascular system during pregnancy include an expansion of blood volume and a decrease in hemoglobin concentration. Administration of an iron preparation supplements the diet to meet the expanded red blood cell needs of the mother and the fetus. The most common side effect of oral iron preparations is gastrointestinal disturbances. When oral preparations cause vomiting or diarrhea, a parenteral iron preparation may be prescribed.

Mucovicidosis (cystic fibrosis) is an autosomal, recessive hereditary disease. The chances are one in four that this disease will appear in the next child. It is important to give complete and accurate information on the risk of recurrence of a genetically transmitted disease.

Accelerated fetal heart rate patterns reflect the activity of the fetus and its response to contractions. The increased rate described in question 31 is most certainly due to a fetal hypoxia. Careful monitoring and accurate interpretations of fetal heart rates throughout labor permit measures to be taken to prevent complications.

Maternal-infant bonding includes eye contact and touching. Instilling eyedrops before the initial interaction between the mother and infant may result in visual distortion in the newborn.

The behavior of an infant who is breast-fed

will reflect how satisfied the infant is. The infant's readiness to breast-feed will be indicated by restlessness.

The release of oxytocin when the infant is breast-feeding increases the severity of the afterpains. A mild analgesic taken within an hour before feeding the infant will minimize the discomfort.

## QUESTIONS 35-39

Health counseling for a woman includes giving information about normal nutrition, nutritional needs during pregnancy, and nutritional needs of the fetus. The diet should be well balanced and contain essential nutrients. The development of the fetus is dependent upon the mother's diet and not upon her reserves. Protein is important in brain growth. Specific nutritional needs throughout pregnancy should be reviewed.

Between the 17th and the 20th week of pregnancy, quickening and the detection of the fetal heartbeat help to confirm the expected delivery date. Knowledge of the development of the fetus is important to making accurate assessments throughout the prenatal period.

Initial prenatal physical assessment in-cludes pelvic measurements. Further assessment may require radiological examination and sonograms. Cephalopelvic disproportion exists when the the fetal head is too large to pass through the pelvis. Measurements are made by x-ray pelvimetry to assess the anterior-posterior diameter of the pelvis, and sonograms are used for measuring the biparietal diameter of the fetal head.

Hyaline membrane disease, also known as respiratory distress syndrome, generally affects a preterm infant. The infant fails to synthesize lecithin at the required rate to prevent alveoli from collapsing. Early detection and aggressive treatment are essential.

## QUESTIONS 40-45

During the first trimester the woman is aware of the physical changes in her body. Breast changes may occur prior to missing the first menses. In addition, early physical changes include amenorrhea, urinary frequency, and gastrointestinal disorders (nausea and vomiting).

The initial prenatal assessment must include information about the woman's nutritional status in order to promote her health and the normal development of fetal organs.

Monitoring weight gain throughout pregnancy is essential in order to control excessive caloric intake and especially to detect excessive fluid retention and possible pregnancy-induced hypertension.

The bluish discoloration of the infant's hands and feet in the first few hours after birth results from poor peripheral circulation, which causes vasomotor instability. Assessment of central circulation should be made by blanching the skin and noting the return of the blood supply.

Whenever a patient is emotionally upset, it is most important for the nurse to indicate interest and willingness to listen, if the patient wishes to talk. Most women experience a transient depression in the early postpartum period. They become tearful, have difficulty sleeping, and experience anorexia. The experience of labor, adjustments following delivery, and hormonal changes are probable causes of the depression.

## QUESTIONS 46-54

Changes noted during the first trimester of pregnancy include urinary frequency. Gradual enlargement of the abdomen begins about the 12th week of gestation, when the fundus of the uterus becomes palpable above the symphysis pubis. Quickening occurs during the second trimester, and lightening occurs at the end of the third trimester, before the onset of labor.

A woman's expression of ambivalence about being pregnant is a common occurrence at the time the pregnancy is suspected or confirmed. Establishing an accepting and trusting relationship that permits expression of feelings by the woman is an important supportive measure.

Nonprescription as well as prescription drugs may cause structural defects during the period of organ development in the fetus. Alcoholic beverages and smoking also have an effect on the fetus.

Taking deep breaths at regular intervals while sedentary for long periods is helpful in promoting respiratory gas exchange, but walking around periodically is most important. Walking will prevent venous stasis in the lower extremities and reduce fatigability.

Following the rupture of the membranes, asessment of fetal heart tones should be performed first. The rupture of the membranes may cause prolapse of the umbilical cord, especially if the head of the fetus is unengaged. Compression of the cord will cause fetal hypoxia.

As the end of labor approaches during the second stage, it is most important to remain with the woman. Support and encouragement is required when the efforts of labor become exhausting.

The initial feeding of most newborns is sterile water. This feeding is used to assess the infant's gag reflex and ability to suck and swallow. Any water aspirated during the assessment will not be damaging to lung tissue. The assessment also assists in detecting esophageal abnormalities.

Parent-child bonding is promoted by physical closeness and eye contact. Teaching is important for the mother who is bottle-feeding her infant to insure the emotional and physical comfort of the infant.

The neurological assessment of the newborn should include testing reflexes. The Moro reflex may be tested by striking the mattress.

A sudden loud noise causes a similar response in the infant. Knowledge of testing reflexes in the newborn is essential.

QUESTIONS 55-60

A female infant will often have a thick, white vaginal discharge that may become blood-tinged. This discharge is normal and should disappear in about a week.

The decreased muscle tone in the uterus of multiparas results in afterpains that cause discomfort. Afterpains are more severe during breast-feeding. Mild analgesics are often prescribed.

To assist a woman whose partner objects to breast-feeding requires obtaining information before determining an approach to the problem. The objections of the partner need to be known first. The nurse's primary responsibility is to support the woman's decision.

In the immediate postpartum period, frequent assessment of the uterus is essential. Displacement of the uterus is often indicative of bladder distention, and measures are required to prevent complications, which include hemorrhage.

Excessive bleeding may be indicative of loss of tone in the uterus; the fundus should be checked first. Bleeding may be the result of other problems and it requires investigation if the uterine fundus is firm.

The technique of breast-feeding that promotes both the mother's and the infant's well-being should be taught early. The correct grasp and release of the nipple by the infant will prevent sore nipples.

## QUESTIONS 61-65

Medical disorders such as diabetes mellitus are directly affected by a pregnancy and the disease or condition may have a direct affect on the outcome of the pregnancy. Modifications in the care of women with medical problems throughout pregnancy is important. The woman's understanding of her disease and pregnancy is most essential. Fetal lung maturity is assessed by obtaining a sample of amniotic fluid by amniocentesis.

The probability of having a cesarean section increases when the woman has diabetes. The primary reason is to prevent fetal death. Close monitoring of the infant after delivery is critical. When the choice is to induce labor by administering oxytocin, precautions should be taken to administer the medication at the prescribed rate and to monitor contractions frequently. Prolonged contractions necessitate giving serious consideration to altering the rate of administration or to discontinuing the drug. The management of a woman receiving oxytocin requires constant observation and assessment. Measures include monitoring vital signs frequently.

Assessment of fetal heart tones should be the first action taken after membranes rupture.

## QUESTIONS 66-82

Ambivalence about being pregnant is a common occurrence. The nurse's response should recognize the ambivalence in an accepting manner.

Nutritional counseling in the antepartal period should include teaching the woman the foods that are highest in essential nutrients. Peanut butter and milk in puddings offer the most protein of the choices given.

When a woman elects to breast-feed her infant, the preparation should begin before the end of the pregnancy. Measures such as rubbing the nipples gently with a towel will toughen the nipple and reduce discomfort when beginning to breast-feed the infant.

Cultural considerations for the pregnant woman should be respected. The nurse should have knowledge of cultural differences that may be important to the woman. When a woman has beliefs about when an infant's clothing should be purchased, the nurse should acknowledge the woman's right to carry out her wishes. It is important for the nurse to add what is known about the status of the fetus.

Estrogen excreted in the urine of a pregnant woman is measured to determine the adequacy of placental function. The level of the hormone will also predict whether the fetus is in jeopardy. Estriol level determinations are commonly used in the management of high-risk patients who have underlying medical problems.

The woman should be instructed about the approaching signs of labor, which include lightening, false labor contractions, and beginning dilatation of the cervix. The information must include developments that should bring her into the hospital without delay. This includes rupture of the membranes.

A brief history is obtained when the woman is admitted to the labor and delivery unit. In the event that anesthesia is used, it is important to know the time of the last meal in order to take measures to prevent aspiration.

As the woman's discomfort increases in the transition phase, she becomes increasingly apprehensive and irritable. She may be hyperventilating and having difficulty following instructions. During this phase, performing breathing exercises with her will provide support by assisting her in maintaining control.

Once the cervix is fully dilated, the second stage of labor for a primigravida should end with the delivery of the infant in about one hour. The administration of an analgesic could affect the infant and result in difficulties in the period following birth.

An episiotomy may be performed to prevent excessive stretching and trauma to the perineum during the delivery. Following repair, measures will be required to reduce pain and swelling.

The Apgar score is used to assess the physical condition of the newborn one minute and five minutes after birth. Data are obtained about the infant's heart rate, respiratory status, muscle tone, response of reflexes, and color.

Methylergonovine maleate is an ergot alkaloid that stimulates smooth muscles to contract, thereby clamping uterine blood vessels and controlling bleeding.

To prevent ophthalmia neonatorum, silver nitrate solution or an antibiotic ointment is administered. It is desirable to permit the infant to establish eye contact with the mother to promote the bonding process before treating the infant's eyes.

After the infant is admitted to the nursery and a complete assessment is performed, it is most important to help the infant maintain normal body temperature by providing warmth.

Early detection and reporting of jaundice is essential. Physiological jaundice does not occur until after 24 hours. It is important to have knowledge of normal findings expected in the newborn.

Taking care of the baby is one of the measures that will promote mother-infant bonding. Rooming-in promotes bonding and helps parents develop their sense of being a family.

For two or three days after delivery, a woman usually displays passive, dependent behavior. After having time to rest and adjust to her recent experience, the woman begins to regain control. A transient depression may follow, during which time the woman may experience anorexia, sleeplessness, and tearfulness. The nurse should offer to remain with the woman if she desires to talk or just to have someone with her.

QUESTIONS 83-90

Nursing goals during a pelvic examination of a woman are to give support, relieve apprehension, and promote relaxation. This is achieved by being present during the examination, giving explanations as the examination is performed, and instructing the woman to take deep breaths slowly through her mouth.

The first prenatal visit should include review of the woman's nutritional status. Most women need to increase their iron intake during pregnancy. Knowledge of foods high in iron, such as oatmeal, is necessary if teaching is to be effective. The total nutritional needs should be reviewed.

Regional anesthesia that interferes with transmission of nerve impulses includes lumbar epidural block. The technique used may be a single injection or a continuous administration of the anesthetic agent through an indwelling catheter. Reactions to the anesthetic agents may be mild or may cause cardiovascular collapse. The reactions usually occur within 5 to 40 minutes, and constant supervision of the woman is essential. Assessment must include monitoring of blood pressure.

Within an hour after delivery, chilling occurs as a normal adjustment to the release of intra-abdominal pressure and the exhaustion associated with the labor process. When chilling occurs, the woman should be covered with a blanket.

The assessment of a newborn requires that care be taken to prevent chilling. Keeping the infant warm is essential.

Interpretation of the results of blood gases confirms the abnormal exchange of respiratory gases. Elevated levels of carbon dioxide and low pH and oxygen content indicate the onset of hypoxia, which should alert the nurse to prepare sodium bicarbonate for administration.

Assessing the character of lochia provides evidence as to whether the involution of the uterus is progressing normally. During the first three days, the lochia should be dark red and may contain a few small clots. By the third day postpartum, the lochia should be pinkish, and it should gradually decrease to a pale yellowish discharge.

Thrush appears as white plaques in the mouth of the newborn and red eruptions on the skin of the diaper area. It is contracted during delivery when the mother has the fungus in the vagina. Thrush may also be seen in susceptible infants who receive long-term antibiotic therapy.

QUESTIONS 91-95

When vaginal bleeding occurs, it is essential to determine the cause in order to protect the fetus by maintaining adequate placental function. Bleeding in the early antepartal period may be due to the onset of a spontaneous abortion. Late in the antepartal period, the bleeding may be due to a placenta previa or an abruptio placentae. Painless vaginal bleeding after the seventh month of gestation is a symptom of placenta previa. Determining the placement of the placenta is essential to determine the risk to the mother and the fetus. Profuse bleeding requires delivery by cesearean section without delay; the woman should therefore be kept fasting.

In the premature infant, there is an absence of subcutaneous fat. Blood vessels can be seen close to the skin surface. To accurately assess the respiratory rate of an infant requires that the infant be at rest.

When a premature infant needs to be transported to a regional center, the mother can be helped to deal with the reality of the situation by having an opportunity to see and touch the infant.

## INDIVIDUAL QUESTIONS 96-100

96. Following an amniocentesis, the woman should be instructed to report the onset of vaginal discharge, abdominal pain, uterine contractions, chills, and fetal hyperactivity or lack of activity.

97. Leg cramps during pregnancy may be related to a phosphorus-calcium imbalance, fatigue, impaired circulation, or pressure of the uterus on nerves.

98. A newborn's temperature may drop to 96.8$^\circ$F. (36.0$^\circ$C.) if the infant is not dried or placed under a radiant warmer in the delivery room. The temperature may also drop as a result of environmental exposure or adaptation to extrauterine life. Further exposure by bathing should be delayed until the infant's temperature has stabilized.

99. When a pregnancy has extended beyond term, it is essential to monitor the fetus for symptoms of placental insufficiency.

100. The umbilical cord normally contains two arteries and one vein. When the cord contains one artery, the infant should be assessed for evidence of congenital anomalies.

# References for Nursing Care During Childbearing

Gilman, Alfred Goodman, et al. The Pharmacological Basis of Therapeutics, 6th ed. New York: Macmillan Publishing Co., 1980.

Jensen, Margaret Duncan, and Irene M. Bobak. Maternity and Gynecologic Care, 3rd ed. St. Louis, MO: The C. V. Mosby Co., 1985.

Krause, Marie V., and Kathleen L. Mahan. Food, Nutrition and Diet Therapy, 7th ed. Philadelphia: W. B. Saunders Co., 1984.

Olds, Sally B., Marcia L. London, and Patricia A. Ladewig. Maternal-Newborn Nursing, A Family-Centered Approach, 2nd ed. Menlo Park, CA: Addison-Wesley Publishing Co., 1984.

Reeder, Sharon J., et al. Maternity Nursing, 15th ed. Philadelphia: J. B. Lippincott Co., 1983.

Rodman, Morton J. and Dorothy W. Smith. Pharmacology and Drug Therapy in Nursing, 2nd ed. Philadelphia: J. B. Lippincott Co., 1979.

Ziegel, Erna E. and Mecca S. Cranley. Obstetric Nursing, 8th ed. New York: Macmillan Publishing Co., 1984.

# NURSING CARE
# OF CHILDREN

Directions: Read each study question carefully. Select one answer from the four choices presented that you think answers the question correctly. There is only one correct answer to each question. Use the answer key to find out whether the answer you selected is the correct one. Read carefully the explanations for the patient situations presented in the study questions, paying particular attention to the explanations for any questions you missed.

Mrs. Anna Brand brings her daughter, Maria, who is 2 months old, to the clinic. Mrs. Brand is informed that Maria should have a diphtheria, tetanus, and pertussis (DTP) immunization at this time.

1. Mrs. Brand asks why Maria needs the DTP immunization at this age. Which of the following information should be given to her?

   A. The possibility of allergic reactions to the diphtheria immunization increases as the child gets older.

   B. The tetanus immunization should be completed before the infant develops the ability to crawl.

   C. There is a high mortality rate in infants who have not been immunized to pertussis.

   D. The immunization will be more effective if it is given before the thymus gland begins to atrophy.

2. Mrs. Brand should be informed that Maria may develop which of these reactions to the DTP immunization?

   A. A slight temperature elevation within the next 24 hours.

   B. A generalized rash on the trunk within the next 2 days.

   C. Redness and swelling at the injection site in 3 or 4 days.

   D. Symptoms of an upper respiratory infection in 5 or 6 days.

3. Mrs. Brand brings Maria to the clinic when she is 6 months old. Mrs. Brand says to the nurse, "I tried feeding Maria a little cereal, but she doesn't like it. She spit it out."

   To assist Mrs. Brand, the nurse should ask her which of these questions?

   A. "Are you placing the cereal toward the back of Maria's tongue?"

   B. "Is the temperature of the cereal you are feeding Maria the same as the temperature of her bottle?"

   C. "Is Maria in an upright sitting position when you feed her the cereal?"

   D. "At what time of day have you been giving Maria the cereal?"

4. When Maria is 2 years old, she has a sickle cell screening test, which is positive. Mrs. Brand should be given which of these interpretations of the test result?

   A. Maria needs immediate supportive therapy.

   B. Maria needs further evaluation to determine her status.

   C. Maria has the sickle cell trait.

   D. Maria has sickle cell anemia.

---
Mrs. Eva Barber brings Susie, 7 years old, and Linda, 8 years old, to the pediatric clinic.
---

5. The nurse gives Susie a book to look at in the waiting room. Susie takes the book without saying anything, and Mrs. Barber indicates that she would like Susie to thank the nurse.

Which of these actions, if taken by Mrs. Barber, would be an effective way of teaching Susie acceptable social behavior?

A. Say to Susie, "It is rude to accept the book without saying thanks."

B. Say to Susie, "I don't know where your manners are today."

C. Say to the nurse, "Thank you for being so thoughtful."

D. Say to the nurse, "Why can't children learn to be polite."

6. Mrs. Barber tells the nurse that Susie has been taking small amounts of money from her purse. She asks, "What should I do about this?" To help Mrs. Barber deal with Susie's behavior, the nurse should suggest that if Susie repeats the behavior, Mrs. Barber should make which of these statements to Susie?

A. "Did you take money from my wallet?"

B. "Where did you learn that when you want money you just take it?"

C. "Taking money without permission is not the way we do things in our family."

D. "You would be unhappy if I took money from your piggy bank."

7. Mrs. Barber says that Susie and Linda occasionally get into fights in which they pull each other's hair. To discourage this type of behavior, the nurse should suggest that Mrs. Barber take which of these actions?

A. Punish the girl who initiated the dispute.

B. Discipline both girls equally.

C. Help the girls to identify each other's positive attributes.

D. Let the girls work out the conflict.

---
Robert Kendall, 2 1/2 years old, has an elevated lead level in his blood and urine. He is admitted to the hospital. His treatment includes a chelating agent, edetate calcium disodium ($CaNa_2EDTA$), intramuscularly.
---

8. The chelating agent for Robert is ordered for which of these purposes?

A. To exchange calcium for lead ions and to promote excretion of the lead through the kidneys.

B. To convert the lead ions into a salt and to promote the production of hemoglobin.

C. To precipitate the lead from the blood and to render it inactive within subcutaneous tissue.

D. To reduce the production of trypsin and to eliminate the lead in the feces.

9. Before Robert is given the first dose of the chelating agent, which of these actions by the nurse is essential?

A. Put Robert in an isolation unit.

B. Take Robert's blood pressure.

C. Weigh Robert.

D. Establish that Robert is voiding sufficient quantities.

10. Without treatment, Robert would be prone to developing the most common sequela to lead poisoning, which is

A. hepatic failure.

B. brain damage.

C. colitis.

D. hypertrophy of the gums.


11. Robert is to receive 240 ml. of intravenous fluids in an 8-hour period. The infusion set delivers 60 drops per ml. He should receive approximately how many drops per minute?

A. 15

B. 30

C. 45

D. 60


12. Robert has all of the following abilities at 2 1/2 years of age. Which one represents his highest level of development?

A. Picking up crumbs using his thumb and index finger.

B. Pointing to a specific body part upon request.

C. Building a tower of eight blocks.

D. Drinking from a cup without assistance.

---
Robert is discharged and returns to the clinic with his mother.
---

13. Mrs. Kendall is upset because Robert is now wetting his bed. He was toilet-trained prior to hospitalization. To respond to Mrs. Kendall, the nurse should use which of these approaches?

A. Explain to Mrs. Kendall that the behavior is expected and that Robert should wear diapers until he adjusts to being at home.

B. Instruct Mrs. Kendall to have Robert void every two hours and suggest that she limit his fluids after dinner.

C. Encourage Mrs. Kendall not to make an issue of Robert's behavior and to praise Robert when he says that he needs to urinate.

D. Tell Mrs. Kendall that bed-wetting is common at Robert's age and that it would be best to ignore his behavior.


14. The nurse discusses nutrition with Mrs. Kendall. Mrs. Kendall says that all of her children seem to dislike vegetables. The nurse should elicit information from Mrs. Kendall that would answer which of these questions?

A. What are the eating habits of Mr. and Mrs. Kendall?

B. Is the financial status of Mr. and Mrs. Kendall sufficient to purchase essential food items?

C. How does Mrs. Kendall prepare meals for the family?

D. Do the children's weights reflect sufficient food intake?

Paula Taft, 1 day old, is admitted to the pediatric intensive care nursery. She has a myelomeningocele that is about 2 in. (5 cm.) in diameter in the lumbosacral area. The covering of the defect is intact. Paula has paralysis of both lower extremities. She is scheduled for surgery the next day.

---

15. The primary objective of preoperative nursing care for Paula should be to prevent

    A. urinary tract infection.

    B. contractures of the hips.

    C. injury to the sac.

    D. accumulation of spinal fluid in the ventricles.

16. The nurse makes all of the following observations of Paula. Which one is most likely related to the myelomeningocele?

    A. Irregular respirations.

    B. Dribbling of urine.

    C. Depressed anterior fontanel.

    D. Mottling of the skin.

---

Paula has the repair of the myelomeningocele. Her postoperative recovery is uncomplicated, and she is discharged in two weeks.

When Paula is 10 weeks old, she is admitted to the hospital because she has developed hydrocephalus. A ventriculoperitoneal shunt is performed, and Paula is transferred from the recovery room to the pediatric unit.

---

17. To assess whether Paula's shunt is functioning, it is most important to include which of these measures in her daily care?

    A. Testing her Moro reflex.

    B. Noting the frequency of her voidings.

    C. Observing her for signs of periorbital edema.

    D. Palpating her anterior fontanel.

---

Richard Uhry, 2 months old, is admitted to the hospital with severe diarrhea of 3 days' duration. Richard has an elevated temperature and he is dehydrated. He is to receive nothing by mouth and is to receive fluids intravenously.

---

18. Richard is to have potassium chloride added to his intravenous fluids. Before adding the potassium, it is essential to make which of these assessments of him?

    A. His pulse rate.

    B. His respiratory rate.

    C. His urinary output.

    D. His pupillary response to light.

19. To prevent circulatory overload in Richard while he is having intravenous therapy, it is essential to take which of these measures?

    A. Changing his position.

    B. Palpating his anterior fontanel.

    C. Checking the specific gravity of his urine.

    D. Monitoring the rate of flow of his infusion.

---

Mark Hall, 2 1/2 years old, has tetralogy of Fallot. He is underweight and of small physical stature. He is admitted to the hospital for palliative surgery.

---

20. Mark has had all of the following conditions since he was 1 year old. Which one is probably most directly related to his small physical size?

    A. Iron deficiency anemia.

    B. Fatigability upon physical exertion.

    C. Frequent periods of wakefulness at night.

    D. Inadequate oxygenation of body tissues.

21. If Mark should have an episode of severe dyspnea prior to surgery, he should be placed in which of these positions?

A. Knee-chest.

B. Sitting upright.

C. Supine.

D. Prone.

---

Billy Jackson, 5 years old, has symptoms suggestive of acute lymphocytic leukemia. Upon admission to the hospital, he has petechiae on his trunk and extremities. Mrs. Jackson plans to stay with Billy.

---

22. Since Billy may have acute leukemia, in addition to the symptoms noted upon Billy's admission, he may also have which of these symptoms?

A. Fatigue.

B. Muscular twitching.

C. Hemoptysis.

D. Bradycardia.

23. Billy is to have a bone marrow aspiration. In preparing him for this procedure, the nurse should consider that a characteristic of 5-year-olds is

A. conforming to parental expectations.

B. understanding simple explanations.

C. being compliant and submissive.

D. responding negatively to verbal directions.

---

The diagnosis of acute lymphocytic leukemia is confirmed. Billy's blood studies include the following results: white blood cell count, 8,500 per cu. mm. ($mm^3$) with abundant blasts; platelet count, 30,000 per cu. mm. ($mm^3$); hemoglobin, 5 gm. per 100 ml.; and hematocrit, 18%.

---

24. Since Billy's platelet count is 30,000 per cu. mm. of blood, it would be most important to include which of these measures in Billy's care plan?

A. Providing him with a soft toothbrush for cleaning his teeth.

B. Offering him fluids that are high in vitamin C.

C. Limiting his contact with other children.

D. Encouraging him to eat foods high in protein.

25. Because of Billy's hemoglobin level, which of these measures should be included in his care?

A. Keeping him on protective isolation.

B. Observing him for dyspnea on exertion.

C. Encouraging him to eat foods that are high in vitamin K.

D. Allowing him to play with toys that are made of soft material.

26. Billy receives a transfusion of packed red cells. Soon after the transfusion is started, Billy says to the nurse, "I'm freezing." Billy is shivering and his teeth are chattering.

The nurse should take which of these actions first?

A. Take Billy's temperature.

B. Obtain a urine specimen from Billy.

C. Explain to Billy that he feels cold because the blood was refrigerated before he received it.

D. Stop Billy's treatment.

27. During the afternoon rest hour, Billy
    starts to sing loudly and jump up and down
    on his bed.  The nurse should take which of
    these actions?

    A. Explain to Billy why he needs to rest.

    B. Play a simple game with Billy.

    C. Give Billy a toy to play with.

    D. Move Billy's bed out into the corridor
       outside his room.

------------------------------------------------
Billy's condition improves and he is to be
discharged.
------------------------------------------------

28. In preparation for Billy's discharge, the
    nurse has a conference with Mrs. Jackson.
    Which of these topics should initially be
    the focus of the conference?

    A. Adapting the hospital treatment plan to
       the home setting.

    B. Providing information about support
       services available to the family.

    C. Reviewing early symptoms Billy will
       develop at the onset of a relapse.

    D. Determining the family's effectiveness
       in coping with Billy's health problem.

29. The nurse should give Mrs. Jackson which of
    these instructions about Billy's activity
    after discharge?

    A. "Billy should be restricted to playing
       with children in the neighborhood."

    B. "Billy should be continuously supervised
       by an adult when he is playing."

    C. "Billy should have scheduled periods of
       rest during the day."

    D. "Billy should be allowed to do anything
       that is suitable for a five-year-old to
       do."

30. Mrs. Jackson tells the nurse that her
    13-year-old daughter seems to fluctuate
    between being able to manage the
    responsibilities of her daily affairs and
    needing help even with the simplest kind of
    decision making.

    Which of these responses by the nurse would
    be most supportive?

    A. "Her behavior is probably a reaction to
       her brother's problem.  Perhaps you
       should consider counseling for her."

    B. "You are describing behavior that is
       typical of thirteen-year-olds.  Let's
       talk about it some more."

    C. "This kind of behavior must be difficult
       for you to handle.  How does she act
       with her father?"

    D. "You are concerned about this behavior.
       How does she behave in school?"

------------------------------------------------
Erica Nadler, 9 years old, is seen in the
clinic for symptoms suggestive of diabetes
mellitus.  Results of tests confirm the
diagnosis.  Erica is to receive isophane (NPH)
insulin every morning.  The nurse has a
conference with Erica and her mother to teach
them about the management of Erica's diabetes.
------------------------------------------------

31. An early indication of Erica's diabetes
    mellitus was most probably which of these
    symptoms?

    A. Anorexia.

    B. Fatigue.

    C. Excessive thirst.

    D. Weight loss.

113

32. When teaching Erica about diabetes mellitus, the nurse should plan an approach that considers that 9-year-olds have which of these characteristics?

    A. Their thinking is based more on fantasy than reality.

    B. Their attention span may be limited.

    C. They can understand cause-and-effect relationships.

    D. They tend to reject parental guidance.

33. Since Erica is to receive NPH insulin every morning, she should be taught to include which of these measures in her care?

    A. Eating a midafternoon snack.

    B. Avoiding strenuous exercise.

    C. Limiting fluid intake after the evening meal.

    D. Scheduling periods of rest throughout the day.

34. When teaching Erica about testing her urine, the nurse should give her which of these instructions about collecting a urine specimen?

    A. "Test a specimen of urine from each voiding throughout the day."

    B. "Collect all urine voided for eight hours, and take a specimen from the total amount to test."

    C. "Start to urinate, stop, and then urinate into a container for the specimen to be tested."

    D. "Empty your bladder, and thirty minutes later urinate again into a container for the specimen to be tested."

35. Erica is taught the symptoms of hypoglycemia, which include

    A. feeling tremulous.

    B. nausea.

    C. headache.

    D. abdominal pain.

------------------------------------------------
A week later, Erica returns to the clinic in the afternoon.
------------------------------------------------

36. While waiting to be seen by the nurse, Erica begins to work on a puzzle. She suddenly throws all the pieces of the puzzle on the floor and seems to be confused. The nurse should take which of these actions first?

    A. Ask Erica to provide a urine specimen.

    B. Determine at what time Erica took her insulin.

    C. Give Erica a glass of sweetened juice to drink.

    D. Question Erica about what is upsetting her.

37. To determine if Erica has ketonuria, the nurse should make which of these assessments?

    A. Determine the sugar content of Erica's urine.

    B. Check the level of Erica's serum glucose.

    C. Test Erica's urine for the presence of acetone.

    D. Measure the specific gravity of Erica's urine.

38. Which of these statements by Erica would indicate that she needs further dietary instruction?

   A. "I don't eat all the vegetables my mother gives me."

   B. "I now buy hard candies instead of chocolates."

   C. "I've started to eat fruit for dessert instead of pastry."

   D. "I eat an extra slice of bread for lunch at school instead of the rice that I hate."

---

Linda Wagner, 8 years old, is admitted to the hospital with pneumonia. Linda has a history of cystic fibrosis and frequent respiratory infections. Her treatment includes inhalation therapy and postural drainage.

---

39. Linda's susceptibility to respiratory infections is directly related to the fact that cystic fibrosis causes which of these physiological alterations?

   A. Formation of mucus plugs in the bronchioles.

   B. Decreased intrapulmonic pressure.

   C. Malformation of the trachea.

   D. Distention of alveoli.

40. The inhalation therapy for Linda is expected to achieve which of these effects first?

   A. To improve the effectiveness of cilia in the respiratory tract.

   B. To increase the use of intercostal muscles in breathing.

   C. To promote the exchange of gases in the alveoli.

   D. To strengthen the movement of the diaphragm.

41. Postural drainage should be scheduled for Linda at which of these times?

   A. Thirty minutes after each meal and at bedtime.

   B. Upon arising, and at midmorning, midafternoon, and bedtime.

   C. Immediately before meals and an hour before bedtime.

   D. Every six hours.

---

Linda is receiving pancreatic enzymes.

---

42. The nurse should have which of these understandings about administering pancreatic enzymes to Linda?

   A. They are given with milk twice a day.

   B. They are given whenever food is ingested.

   C. They are given within an hour after each meal.

   D. They are given with water about an hour before each meal.

43. Linda is given pancreatic enzymes for which of these purposes?

   A. To decrease the peristalsis in the small bowel.

   B. To improve the digestion of fat and protein.

   C. To stimulate secretions of the head of the pancreas.

   D. To reduce the production of endogenous pancreatic secretions.

Linda's condition improves, and she is being
prepared for discharge.

44. Since Linda has respiratory problems
    related to cystic fibrosis, her mother
    should be given which of these instructions
    about Linda's care?

    A. "Linda's use of salt should be limited."

    B. "Linda's fluid intake should be
       restricted to warm drinks."

    C. "Linda should not be given cough
       medication."

    D. "Linda should have a nap every
       afternoon."

45. Linda's mother tells the nurse that she is
    pregnant and she is concerned about the
    possibility that her second child may have
    cystic fibrosis.  Since cystic fibrosis is
    transmitted as an autosomal recessive
    trait, the nurse should give Mrs. Wagner
    which of the following information about
    the chance that other children born to her
    and her husband may have either the trait
    or the disease?

    A. Each child has a 25% chance of having
       the trait and a 50% chance of having the
       disease.

    B. Each child has a 50% chance of having
       the trait and a 25% chance of having the
       disease.

    C. Each child has a 50% chance of having
       the trait and a 50% chance of having the
       disease.

    D. Not enough information is stated to
       determine the chance that other children
       may have the trait or the disease.

Andrew Dunn, 3 1/2 years old, is brought to the
pediatric clinic by his mother because for the
past two days Andrew has been crying whenever he
urinates.  A diagnosis of a urinary tract infection is made, and Andrew is to receive
sulfisoxazole acetyle (Gantrisin Pediatric
Suspension).

46. Considering Andrew's problem and treatment,
    it would be most important to give Mrs.
    Dunn which of these instructons?

    A. "Take Andrew's temperature each day when
       he gets up in the morning and during the
       late afternoon."

    B. "Avoid giving Andrew foods that are high
       in salt, such as potato chips and salted
       crackers."

    C. "Have Andrew drink a small glass of
       water about every hour while he is
       awake."

    D. "Measure Andrew's urine each time he
       voids."

During the next four months, Andrew has
recurrent urinary tract infections.  Andrew is
admitted to the hospital for diagnostic studies
which include a cystoscopic examination.

47. Andrew is to have an intramuscular
    injection before the cystoscopic
    examination.  The nurse can best assist
    Andrew in accepting the injection by using
    which of these approaches?

    A. Tell him what is to be done and how he
       can help the nurse.

    B. Tell him that the injection will not
       hurt very much if he will lie still.

    C. Tell him why the nurse expects him to
       act like a big boy while the injection
       is being given.

    D. Tell him that he will be given a
       lollipop or a cookie afterward if he is
       a good boy while he gets his injection.

48. When Andrew has a need to void for the first time after the cystoscopy, the nurse should take which of these actions?

A. Leave a urinal within his reach.

B. Offer him a urinal after checking that his bladder is palpable.

C. Start him on 24-hour urine collection.

D. Take him to the bathroom to void.

49. The morning after the cystoscopy, Andrew's temperature is 103°F. (39.4°C.). On the basis of all the information provided about Andrew, which of these statements about cystoscopy is pertinent to the cause of Andrew's fever?

A. Cystoscopy may produce an antigen-antibody reaction.

B. Cystoscopy may be an emotionally disturbing procedure.

C. Cystoscopy may precipitate the recurrence of a urinary tract infection.

D. Cystoscopy may cause severe electrolyte imbalance in a 4-year-old.

---

Results of studies reveal that Andrew has a right hydroureter. He has a reimplantation of his right ureter. He is now a week postoperative and is ambulatory.

---

50. Andrew spends most of each day in the playroom. Because of Andrew's age, which of these play materials would be most appropriate for him?

A. A basin of water and plastic cups.

B. A pull toy and a nest of boxes.

C. A ball and jacks.

D. A large colorful ball and a wooden paddle.

---

Andrew is discharged and attends the clinic regularly. He is to have the Denver Developmental Screening Test (DDST) and vision screening.

---

51. In preparation for administering the DDST, the nurse is to calculate Andrew's age. Today is June 10, 1986, and Andrew's birthdate is December 20, 1981. Therefore his age is

A. 4 years, 5 months, 20 days.

B. 4 years, 6 months, 10 days.

C. 5 years, 5 months, 10 days.

D. 5 years, 6 months, 20 days.

52. After the nurse completes the DDST evaluation of Andrew, it would be appropriate to ask Mrs. Dunn which of these questions?

A. "Was Andrew's performance typical of his usual behavior?"

B. "Do you want to know if Andrew scored within the normal range?"

C. "Would you like to discuss the relationship between this test and Andrew's intelligence?"

D. "Do you want Andrew to repeat the test to see if he can do better?"

53. Andrew says to the nurse, "I have a bear that sleeps under my bed. I take him for a walk every day." Which of these responses should the nurse make?

A. "What does the bear eat?"

B. "Do your mother and father know about the bear?"

C. "Tell me the bear's name."

D. "That's a nice story you made up about a bear."

Sharon Gates, 10 years old, is hospitalized with acute rheumatic fever. She has a carditis with congestive heart failure. Steroid therapy and a moderately sodium-restricted diet are ordered for her.

54. Sharon had several tests to establish the diagnosis of rheumatic fever. Which of these tests are commonly used in establishing a diagnosis of rheumatic fever?

    A. Cephalin flocculation, Widal, and blood culture.

    B. Streptococcus MG agglutination, plasma mucoprotein level, and complement fixation.

    C. Latex fixation, throat culture, and complete blood count.

    D. Erythrocyte sedimentation rate, C-reactive protein, and antistreptolysin O titer.

55. During the acute phase of Sharon's illness, her care plan should include

    A. encouraging her active participation in her own care.

    B. limiting her intake of fluids.

    C. restricting foods high in protein.

    D. providing scheduled rest periods.

56. Sharon likes all of the following foods. Mrs. Gates is to bring one of them to Sharon for an evening snack. Because it is LOWEST in sodium, which food should the nurse suggest that Mrs. Gates bring?

    A. Cheeseburger.

    B. Chocolate malted milk.

    C. Orange sherbet.

    D. Slice of pizza.

57. Sharon develops a "moon face" as a result of steroid therapy. One day, the nurse finds her looking in the mirror and crying. When questioned, Sharon says, "I'm ugly!" Which of these understandings about 10-year-olds would help the nurse to meet Sharon's needs at this time?

    A. The depression that occurs in children of Sharon's age as a side effect of steroid therapy usually disappears when therapy is discontinued.

    B. Hospitalized children of Sharon's age react to oversolicitousness by parents and friends.

    C. Many 10-year-olds are concerned with body image, and noticeable deviations from the norm are distressing to them.

    D. The boredom experienced by hospitalized 10-year-olds leads to preoccupation with themselves.

58. Sharon improves and is allowed increased activity. The nurse should initiate which of these plans at this time?

    A. Arrange for the visiting schoolteacher to come to see Sharon.

    B. Ask Mrs. Gates to buy Sharon a new toy that will require physical activity.

    C. Consult with the play therapist to determine ways for Sharon to have stimulating social experiences while she is in the hospital.

    D. Have each team member spend a designated amount of time with Sharon daily.

59. To prevent recurrent attacks of rheumatic fever, which of these plans will be recommended for Sharon?

    A. Limited contacts with young children.

    B. A diet of high caloric value.

    C. A schedule that provides specific rest periods.

    D. Prophylactic drug therapy.

Mrs. Roberts brings her son, Edward, to the well-child clinic on a regular basis. Edward is now 4 months old.

60. Mrs. Roberts says that she is giving Edward some solid foods. The nurse discusses the practice of introducing new foods separately to an infant. The nurse should give which of these rationales for this practice?

A. The sense of smell will be sharpened.

B. Taste buds will develop sensitivity.

C. Food likes and dislikes will be easier to identify.

D. Allergic reactions, if any, will be more readily detected.

61. Edward demonstrates the following behaviors. If his growth and development have been following a normal pattern, which behavior did he most likely learn last?

A. Smiling at his mirror image.

B. Rolling from his abdomen to his side.

C. Raising his head and shoulders from the prone position.

D. Looking at his hands while holding them in front of him.

62. When Edward is 8 months old, Mrs. Roberts makes all of the following comments to the nurse. Which one should definitely be investigated?

A. "Edward frequently gets up on his knees and rocks himself until he falls asleep."

B. "Lately Edward won't go to sleep unless there's a night-light on in his room."

C. "Edward has a hard time going to sleep unless he takes a bottle of juice to bed with him."

D. "Edward usually wakes up an hour after he goes to sleep, cries for a few minutes, and then goes back to sleep."

Mrs. Bader, who lives next to a hospital, dashes into the emergency room with her 2 1/2-year-old son, Daniel. Mrs. Bader tells the nurse that she found Daniel playing with an empty bottle of baby aspirin and that there are pieces of aspirin in his mouth and on his lips. The aspirin bottle had been about half full.

63. The nurse takes Mrs. Bader and Daniel to an examining room. The nurse should take which of these actions next?

A. Stimulate Daniel's gag reflex.

B. Administer 60 ml. of mineral oil to Daniel.

C. Give Daniel 10 ml. of an antacid preparation.

D. Obtain a urine specimen from Daniel.

64. The nurse should observe Daniel for symptoms of salicylate poisoning, which include

A. diplopia.

B. photophobia.

C. hyperventilation.

D. facial flushing.

65. Daniel is given vitamin $K_1$ intramuscularly. The purpose of this drug for him is to

A. stimulate platelet production.

B. counteract possible hypoprothrombinemia.

C. prevent hemolysis of red blood cells.

D. promote bone marrow activity.

---
Debra Vinson, 9 months old, is brought to the clinic by her mother. An examination and blood tests reveal that Debra has anemia and otitis media.
---

66. The nurse obtains all of the following information from Mrs. Vinson. Which information is probably most directly related to Debra's having anemia?

A. Mrs. Vinson's husband lost his job two months ago.

B. Mrs. Vinson had a spontaneous miscarriage four months before she became pregnant with Debra.

C. Mrs. Vinson was delivered of Debra two months prematurely.

D. Mrs. Vinson gained ten pounds during her pregnancy.

67. To confirm the diagnosis of anemia, Debra most probably had which of these diagnostic tests performed?

A. Bone marrow aspiration.

B. Gastric analysis.

C. Leukocyte count.

D. Hematocrit determination.

68. Debra is to be given nose drops. To promote the most therapeutic effect from the nose drops, the nurse should take which of these measures?

A. Giving the medication about a half hour before Debra is fed.

B. Diluting the medication with normal saline before giving it to Debra.

C. Placing Debra in Trendelenburg position after the drops are given.

D. Suctioning the secretions in Debra's nostrils after the drops are given.

69. The next day the physician considers a myringotomy for Debra. The procedure is performed for which of these purposes?

A. To promote drainage from the ear.

B. To irrigate the eustachian tube.

C. To equalize pressure on the tympanic membrane.

D. To correct a congenital malformation in the inner ear.

70. Mrs. Vinson informs the nurse that Debra has refused solid food and that her diet has consisted mostly of milk and simple carbohydrates. To ensure that Debra receives necessary nutrients, the nurse should recommend which of these measures to Debra's mother?

A. Withholding desserts from Debra until she has eaten the vegetables served to her.

B. Mixing strained food into the milk that is given to Debra.

C. Having Debra eat small amounts of meat and vegetables before offering her milk.

D. Excluding milk from Debra's diet until she begins to like other foods served to her.

---
Eric Greene, 3 months old, is admitted to the hospital for repair of a right inguinal hernia.
---

71. An inguinal hernia in infants such as Eric is usually repaired as soon as possible after the diagnosis is made. The primary purpose is to prevent

A. intussusception.

B. incarceration.

C. gonadal hypertrophy.

D. thickening of the spermatic cord.

72. Mrs. Greene tells the nurse that when she learned that Eric would require surgery to repair the inguinal hernia, she began to give him twice the prescribed amount of a multivitamin preparation. The nurse's response should be based on which of these understandings about the possible effect of Mrs. Greene's action?

A. An overdose of fat-soluble vitamins may be toxic.

B. Megadoses of vitamins before a surgical procedure may prevent depletion of vitamins in the early postoperative period.

C. Large amounts of water-soluble vitamins may alter the autoimmune system.

D. Increased quantities of vitamins may accelerate growth.

---

Eric has the surgical repair of the right inguinal hernia. His postoperative recovery is good. He is to be discharged.

---

73. Before Eric is discharged, he is to receive an immunization intramuscularly. The nurse should administer the intramuscular injection into which of these muscles?

A. Biceps.

B. Dorsogluteal.

C. Vastus lateralis.

D. Ventrogluteal.

---

Bobby Young, 22 months old, is admitted to the hospital with acute laryngotracheobronchitis. He is to be placed in a mist tent with compressed air.

---

74. Bobby is placed in the mist tent for which of these purposes?

A. To inhibit the production of surfactant.

B. To increase the surface tension of the mucous membranes of the respiratory tract.

C. To increase oxygen and carbon dioxide exchange.

D. To provide an environment that will decrease the rate of growth of pathogenic organisms.

75. All of the following goals may be included in Bobby's nursing care. During the acute period of his illness, which one should have priority?

A. To provide optimum nutrition.

B. To conserve his energy.

C. To maintain the integrity of his skin.

D. To stimulate his senses.

76. Which of these symptoms in Bobby would be an early sign of hypoxia?

A. Mouth breathing.

B. Flushing of the face.

C. Barking cough.

D. Increased restlessness.

David Folles, 5 weeks old, is admitted to the hospital for a pyloromyotomy for pyloric stenosis. His preoperative orders include atropine sulfate.

---

77. Which of these symptoms was an early indication that David had pyloric stenosis?

    A. Diarrhea.

    B. Dehydration.

    C. Regurgitation.

    D. Abdominal distention.

78. David is to receive 0.15 mg. of atropine. To prepare the medication, the nurse uses a vial containing 0.4 mg. of atropine in 1 ml. of solution. To administer the prescribed dose to David, the nurse should give him how many milliliters of the solution?

    A. 0.30

    B. 0.34

    C. 0.38

    D. 0.42

79. If David has a reaction to atropine, the nurse would observe which of these symptoms?

    A. Lethargy.

    B. Tremors.

    C. Restlessness.

    D. Flushed skin.

David has the pyloromyotomy as scheduled. He progresses rapidly and is discharged. When David is 4 months old, he is seen in the well-baby clinic.

---

80. The nurse obtains all of the following information from an assessment of David's development. Which information most clearly indicates that the desired effects of the surgical procedure have been achieved?

    A. He weighs twice his birth weight.

    B. He makes sounds in response to attention.

    C. He is irritable when his sleep is disturbed.

    D. He is showing increased drooling.

---

Janice Codden, 7 years old, is admitted to the hospital with a possible acute appendicitis.

---

81. Since it is suspected that Janice has acute appendicitis, it would be most important to obtain the answer to which of these questions?

    A. When did Janice last void?

    B. When did Janice last eat?

    C. When did Janice begin to have pain?

    D. When did Janice have a physical examination?

82. Janice complains of abdominal pain. To relieve some of her discomfort, she should be assisted to assume which of these positions?

    A. Supine.

    B. Prone.

    C. Trendelenburg.

    D. Mid-Fowler's.

83. Janice has blood studies done. Which of these test results, if elevated, would be indicative of acute appendicitis?

A. Hematocrit.

B. Leukocyte count.

C. Erythrocyte count.

D. Serum protein.

84. Janice asks the nurse, "Is the doctor going to cut me? That will hurt." The nurse's response should include which of these statements?

A. "It is not definite that you will have surgery. I will tell you about it when the decision is made."

B. "The doctor may have to cut you. The pain will be gone and you will go home in a few days."

C. "Tell me what you know about the appendix. You must have a friend who had the same problem that you do."

D. "A small incision is made to remove the appendix. You will not feel pain because you will be asleep during the surgery."

-------------------------------------------------
Bonnie Fields, 15 years old, is admitted to the hospital after she ingested an unknown number of barbiturate capsules. Her parents found her on the bathroom floor with an empty bottle by her side. Bonnie is stuporous.
-------------------------------------------------

85. Bonnie's initial care should give priority to which of these measures?

A. Catheterizing her to obtain a urine specimen.

B. Maintaining the patency of her airway.

C. Assessing her level of consciousness.

D. Initiating intravenous therapy for her.

86. An improvement in Bonnie's condition would be indicated most reliably by which of these observations?

A. Her pupils constrict in response to light.

B. Her average hourly urine output is 40 ml. an hour.

C. Her eyes open when her name is called.

D. Her skin feels warm and dry to the touch.

87. The next morning Bonnie is alert and responsive. She does not make any reference to the reason for her hospitalization. The nurse should take which of these actions?

A. Remain readily available to Bonnie in case she wants to talk.

B. Discuss with Bonnie the high incidence of suicide among teenagers.

C. Ask Bonnie to explain her feelings when she took the barbiturates.

D. Explain to Bonnie that therapists are available to help her solve her problems.

-------------------------------------------------
Roger Winter, 13 years old, was riding his bicycle when he was struck by a car. He is brought to the emergency room by ambulance. He has a fracture of his left midthigh and possible head injuries. His mother is summoned, and he is given emergency treatment before being admitted to the hospital.
-------------------------------------------------

88. Considering the nature of Roger's injuries, which of the following information about his history will be most important?

A. When did Roger last eat solid food?

B. Has Roger ever had a tetanus booster?

C. Has Roger had a previous hospitalization?

D. Can Roger recall how the accident happened?

89. Roger's left leg is placed in skeletal traction. The primary purpose of this measure for him is to

A. promote bone healing.

B. align the ends of the fractured bone.

C. reduce pain.

D. control bleeding into the tissues.


90. The results of skull x-rays indicate that Roger may have a fractured skull. It is essential that the nurse observe him for which of these symptoms?

A. Ecchymosis around the eyes.

B. Periorbital edema.

C. Complaints of frontal headache.

D. Evidence of spinal fluid in the nose and ears.


91. After two days of observation, Roger's condition is good. A long leg cast is applied to his left leg. Following the application of the cast, it is most important that Roger's care include which of these measures?

A. Keeping Roger's affected leg elevated on pillows.

B. Assessing Roger's pedal pulses.

C. Placing a cotton blanket over Roger's casted extremity.

D. Supporting Roger's midcalf and midthigh when repositioning the casted extremity.


---
Roger is to be discharged. Follow-up care will be given in the clinic.
---

92. Before Roger is discharged, he should be given which of the following information about the care of his affected extremity?

A. "Reinforce the cast with adhesive tape if any cracks occur."

B. "Having your friends sign their names on your cast may create pressure points on your leg."

C. "Be careful not to spill any liquids on your cast."

D. "Ignore any crumbling of the cast that may occur around the edges."


---
The remainder of the questions are individual questions.
---

93. When admitting to the hospital a child who is mentally retarded, which of these measures would be more important for this child than for a child of average intelligence?

A. Asking the parents for information about the child's level of abilities.

B. Explaining to the parents how continuity of care is given to each child.

C. Orienting the child and the parents to the unit.

D. Discussing routines of diagnostic tests with the parents and the child.

94. John Rand, 2 years old, has a positive reaction to a tuberculin skin test (Mantoux). Which of these interpretations of this finding is correct?

A. John has developed immunity to tuberculosis as a result of the body's reaction to maternal antibodies.

B. John has been infected with the tubercle bacillus.

C. John has developed resistance to the tubercle bacillus.

D. John may have had a respiratory infection recently that has caused a false positive reaction.


95. A newborn has esophageal atresia with a tracheoesophageal fistula. Symptoms characteristic of this condition include

A. frequent, loose stools and constant hunger.

B. visible peristalsis in the upper abdomen and cyanosis.

C. refusal to take water or formula and sternal retraction.

D. choking when being fed and excessive drooling.


96. Gretchen Adams, 3 years old, is brought to the emergency room by her mother. Gretchen has been vomiting. The nurse makes all of the following observations of Gretchen. Which one should lead the nurse to suspect that Gretchen is an abused child?

A. Gretchen's weight is at the 60th percentile and her height is at the 70th percentile for her age.

B. Gretchen has recent abrasions on her knees.

C. One section of Gretchen's hair is cut close to her scalp.

D. When a venipuncture is done, Gretchen lies motionless.


97. The nurse makes all of the following observations of mothers in a well-child clinic. Which behavior is characteristic of mothers who abuse their children?

A. The mother of a 4-month-old girl says to her, "Oh, you just spit up on Mommy's dress. I thought you were through with that."

B. The mother of an 8-month-old boy who is pulling her hair says to him, "Ouch, that hurts."

C. The mother of a 2-year-old boy slaps his hand once after he throws a paper cup on the floor.

D. The mother of a 14-month-old girl says to another mother, "She is so stubborn. I just can't get her toilet-trained."


98. Anthony Kass, a 7-year-old with hemophilia, has his leg splinted following a hemorrhage into the knee joint. The day after the leg is splinted, Anthony complains of increased pain in the affected knee.

On the basis of the information provided, the most justifiable explanation of the pain experienced by Anthony is that it is due to

A. infection.

B. increased bleeding.

C. muscle hypertrophy.

D. friction between adjacent articular joint surfaces.

99. Rebecca Lyons, 10 years old, is receiving phenytoin (Dilantin) sodium following a grand mal seizure. Rebecca should be observed for side effects of Dilantin therapy, which include

A. irritability.

B. frontal headaches.

C. gingival hypertrophy.

D. leukocytosis.

100. Wanda Bill, 13 years old, comes to the adolescent clinic for the first time. While taking Wanda's health history, the nurse learns that Wanda had her first menstrual period 6 months ago and has had only two menstrual periods since then.

The nurse's interpretation of this information should be based on which of these understandings about menarche and menstrual irregularity?

A. Following the onset of menarche, menstrual periods are commonly irregular.

B. True menarche is often preceded by episodes of vaginal spotting, which can be mistaken for menstrual periods.

C. Irregular menstrual periods for more than a few months following menarche indicate difficulty in accepting female identity.

D. Anemia is the primary cause of irregular menstrual cycles in the period immediately following menarche.

This is the end of the study questions for Nursing Care of Children. Check to see whether you selected the correct answer to each question by using the answer key on page 127. Explanations for the correct answers in each patient situation begin on page 128. Read the explanations carefully, paying particular attention to the explanations for any questions you answered incorrectly. Then select a reference book from the list of recommended texts on page 138. Read the section that pertains to each patient situation presented in the study questions.

# Answer Key to Study Questions
## for Nursing Care of Children

| | | | | |
|---|---|---|---|---|
| 1. C | 21. A | 41. B | 61. A | 81. B |
| 2. A | 22. A | 42. B | 62. C | 82. D |
| 3. A | 23. B | 43. B | 63. A | 83. B |
| 4. B | 24. A | 44. C | 64. C | 84. D |
| 5. C | 25. B | 45. B | 65. B | 85. B |
| 6. C | 26. D | 46. C | 66. C | 86. C |
| 7. D | 27. B | 47. A | 67. D | 87. A |
| 8. A | 28. D | 48. D | 68. A | 88. B |
| 9. D | 29. D | 49. C | 69. A | 89. B |
| 10. B | 30. B | 50. B | 70. C | 90. D |
| 11. B | 31. C | 51. A | 71. B | 91. B |
| 12. C | 32. C | 52. A | 72. A | 92. C |
| 13. C | 33. A | 53. D | 73. C | 93. A |
| 14. A | 34. D | 54. D | 74. C | 94. B |
| 15. C | 35. A | 55. D | 75. B | 95. D |
| 16. B | 36. C | 56. C | 76. D | 96. D |
| 17. D | 37. C | 57. C | 77. C | 97. D |
| 18. C | 38. B | 58. A | 78. C | 98. B |
| 19. D | 39. A | 59. D | 79. D | 99. D |
| 20. D | 40. A | 60. D | 80. A | 100. A |

# Explanations for Study Questions
## for Nursing Care of Children

QUESTIONS 1-4

The recommended schedule for immunization is information nurses need in order to counsel families with children. The optimum age for immunization is also important. Immunization to pertussis is recommended for children under 6 years of age. There is a high mortality rate in infants who are not immunized to pertussis. It is not given to children over 6 years of age, because beyond that age the risk of receiving the vaccine increases while the mortality rate of the disease decreases.

Reactions to routine immunizations are usually minor. Side effects of pertussis immunization are usually a temperature elevation and a local reaction at the injection site within 24 to 48 hours.

An initial feeding of solid food, if placed well back in the mouth, will be more easily retained and swallowed.

When the result of a sickle cell screening test is positive, it is necesssary to perform a hemoglobin electrophoresis to establish whether the child has the trait or the disease.

QUESTIONS 5-7

A 7-year-old child begins to be more sensi-

tive and will respond to behavior demonstrated by adults. Therefore, it is important to teach by setting an example. Because children of this age seek family approval, their behavior may be corrected by indicating that undesired behavior is not acceptable in the family. Disputes between siblings of this age are usually more verbal than physical. They should be left to work out their own conflict. Knowledge of the general characteristics of school-age children is necessary in order to assess their developmental level.

QUESTIONS 8-14

Lead poisoning generally occurs as a result of ingesting products containing lead, such as lead-based paint. Some children between 18 and 30 months of age have a compulsive habit of eating nonfood substances. Screening procedures identify those children with serum lead levels that require chelating therapy. The treatment removes lead from blood and tissues by combining it with calcium and promoting its excretion through the kidneys. Monitoring fluid intake and output is not important.

Untreated lead poisoning can result in anemia and kidney damage, but the most serious damage occurs in the brain.

The administration of fluids requires accurate calculation of the drop rate to insure infusion at the prescribed rate. Circulatory overload must be prevented. Frequent monitoring of the drop rate is essential, as is assessment of the condition of the insertion site. The correct drop rate for the situation presented is 30 drops per minute.

At 2 1/2 years of age, building a tower of blocks represents the highest level of development. At 1 year, a child is able to pick up crumbs; at 15 months drink from a cup with little difficulty; and at 18 months, point to body parts.

A stressful experience, such as hospitalization, may cause a toddler to revert to bedwetting. Parents should be encouraged to be patient and to praise the child who is ready to make known his need to urinate.

The food preferences and eating habits of children are influenced by the habits of the parents as well as the developmental level of the child.

## QUESTIONS 15-17

A myelomeningocele is a protrusion of a sac-like cyst of meninges, spinal fluid, and a portion of the spinal cord through a structural defect in the vertebral column. Initial care involves preventing rupture of the sac and its potential for infection. Early surgical repair is required. A myelomeningocele is a frequent cause of neurogenic bladder disfunction and may require a system of bladder drainage.

The child with a myelomeningocele usually has a concurrent hydrocephalus that is treated by a ventriculoperitoneal shunt. Following surgery, tenseness and bulging of the anterior fontanel would be indicative of a malfunction of the shunt.

## QUESTIONS 18-19

Dehydration for any cause may be a life-threatening situation in infants. Initial therapy is directed toward restoring extra-cellular fluid volume. In the presence of acidosis, sodium bicarbonate will probably be administered. When renal function is restored, potassium will be added. Monitoring of serum electrolytes is important. It is essential to maintain the prescribed rate of flow to prevent circulatory overload while assessing the infant's response to treatment.

## QUESTIONS 20-21

Children with tetralogy of Fallot have episodes of cyanosis and hypoxia. They have delayed physical growth and development. Chronic hypoxia may cause mental slowness. The child learns to limit his own physical activity and that squatting relieves hypoxia. When lying down, he assumes a knee-chest position to relieve dyspnea.

The toddler engages in parallel play and considers toys to be his possessions. He is also beginning to learn socialized behavior, which can be reinforced by increasing his awareness of others, such as asking him what toy he would like to give to another child.

QUESTIONS 22-30

The symptoms of acute lymphocytic leukemia include fever, pallor, fatigue, anorexia, petechiae and bone pain.

A 5-year-old who is being prepared for a procedure should be given a simple explanation. He is capable of understanding explanations, and questions should be answered directly and matter-of-factly.

A low platelet count will cause bleeding, and measures need to be taken to prevent injury to soft tissue, such as providing a soft toothbrush. A decreased erythrocyte count causes anemia. This reduces the body's oxygen-carrying capability, and slight exertion may cause dyspnea.

Sudden shaking chills soon after a blood transfusion is started may be an indication of a hemolytic reaction, and the transfusion should be discontinued without delay. The blood should be saved to retype and cross-match. The child's vital signs should be monitored frequently, and a urine specimen should be obtained for analysis.

To promote rest between periods of activity, the nurse should involve the child in a quiet activity, such as a simple game. Although the child at 5 years of age is capable of understanding an explanation about his need for rest, he will not always feel the need to comply.

Before a child with a serious illness is discharged from the hospital, it is important to assess the parent's ability to cope with the situation. Further instruction or referrals may be necessary to provide required support. Following discharge, when the child is in remission from the disease, he should be permitted to function as a normal child of his age, in order to promote his normal growth and development. Therapies used in the treatment of acute leukemia should be reviewed.

The pubertal changes in young adolescents are accompanied by bewilderment, which often leads to inconsistent and unpredictable behavior. Their families need to provide love and support during this maturation process.

QUESTIONS 31-38

An outstanding symptom of diabetes mellitus in children is thirst. Early symptoms that are not usually suspected to be related to diabetes are irritability, fatigue, and bed-wetting. Weight loss may occur, but it is usually gradual and not noticed by parents. Other symptoms often differ from those of adults who have non-insulin-dependent diabetes. These differences should be reviewed.

When a 9-year-old is being taught about diabetes, the child should be given accurate information explaining the cause-and-effect relationship, which a 9-year-old can understand.

Any person taking NPH insulin should be instructed that a midafternoon snack may be required. This time precedes the expected onset of the peak action of NPH insulin.

Urine testing may be included in the daily management of diabetes. In order to obtain a fresh specimen, specimens of urine should be obtained about a half hour after completely emptying the bladder. Testing methods for determining the glucose content of blood and urine should be taught to patients.

Symptoms of hypoglycemia have a rapid onset. The child's behavior will suddenly change and the child will have feelings of tremulousness. A carbohydrate, such as sweetened juice, should be given before obtaining a urine specimen or performing an assessment. Testing urine for the presence of acetone would determine ketonuria.

Dietary instruction is very important. The basics of normal nutrition for a child should be reviewed. The diet should meet the requirements of normal growth and development as well as the requirements imposed by the diabetes. Knowledge of the basic foods and appropriate exchanges is required. Simple carbohydrates in any form are not advised for the diet of a person with diabetes. An important aspect of teaching for the child is learning how to respond when peer influence may be exerted in social situations.

QUESTIONS 39-45

The susceptibility to pneumonia is caused by the viscosity of mucus gland secretions in the respiratory tract. Treatment includes inhalation therapy in an effort to reduce the viscosity of secretions and to promote the action of cilia. Postural drainage facilitates the removal of secretions. The procedure should be performed upon arising, midway between meals, and at bedtime. The child needs time to rest after the procedure, so the procedure should be scheduled so as not to interfere with mealtimes.

Children with cystic fibrosis do not have the pancreatic enzymes necessary for the digestion of protein, fat, and complex carbohydrates. Replacement therapy is required, and pancreatic enzymes are given whenever food is taken. The dosage is regulated in order to obtain normal bowel movements.

Discharge teaching includes measures to promote elimination of respiratory secretions. It is therefore important to avoid the use of cough medication that will suppress coughing.

Fluids should be encouraged. Children with cystic fibrosis have an excess of sodium and chloride in saliva and sweat. They should be encouraged to add salt to their food. Excessive fatigue should be avoided, but scheduled rest periods are not required.

Cystic fibrosis is inherited as an autosomal recessive trait. The defective gene is inherited from both parents. Each child has a 50% chance of having the trait and a 25% chance of having the disease.

## QUESTIONS 46-53

Treatment of a urinary tract infection with sulfonimides requires increasing fluid intake to prevent crystal formation in the urine.

Recurrent urinary tract infections require diagnostic tests to determine the presence of anatomic abnormalities. Cystoscopic examinations for young children are often done under general anesthesia. Simple, straightforward statements of what is to be done should be used to explain procedures to children 3 to 4 years old. The procedure may also be explained by using a doll.

After the cystoscopy, when the child has the need to void, he should be taken to the bathroom. Occasionally, the cystoscopic examination may precipitate a recurrence of an infection, with resulting temperature elevation and possible chills, flank pain, and vomiting.

Appropriate toys for the normal developmental level of a 3-to-4 year-old are a pull toy and a nest of boxes.

The Denver Developmental Screening Test is used to assess the developmental level of children from birth through 6 years of age. When the test is administered, the parent should be asked if the child's behavior during the test was typical of his usual behavior.

Imaginary playmates are an integral part of a preschooler's life. During play, fantasy and reality are not distinguishable to the child. Adults should accept the child's expression of fantasy, but their response should indicate that it is known to be a fantasy.

## QUESTIONS 54-59

Acute rheumatic fever is an inflammatory disease that occurs primarily in school-age children who have had an untreated group A streptococcal infection. Rheumatic fever affects the heart, joints, central nervous system, and subcutaneous tissue.

The diagnostic test that supports objective evidence of rheumatic fever is antistreptolysin O titer. Supporting data is provided by an elevated erythrocyte sedimentation rate, presence of C-reactive protein, leukocytosis, and electrocardiogram tracings.

Encouragement of bed rest is essential to give time for the heart to heal. Treatment also includes salicylates for relief of joint pain; antibiotic therapy, with penicillin the drug of choice; a sodium-restricted diet when indicated; and steroid therapy if congestive

heart failure develops.

When side effects of steroid therapy, such as a "moon face" develop, a 10-year-old may be concerned with body image. It is important to be supportive of the child and to explain the temporary nature of the effect of steroids.

Once the child is permitted increased activity, it is important to initiate school-work. This provides the child with meaningful activity, prevents boredom, and controls the level of energy expenditure.

Continued care after discharge is important. Parents should be taught to take the child's vital signs. Daily rest periods and isolation from persons with acute upper respiratory infections are urged. Prophylactic treatment with penicillin will continue for a long period.

## QUESTIONS 60-62

The schedule for introduction of solid food to infants should be followed. One new food is introduced at a time so that any allergic response may be detected immediately. New foods should be introduced at intervals of several days.

Normal growth and development patterns indicate that smiling at his mirror image is the most recently learned behavior. Rolling from the abdomen to the side occurs by 16 weeks of age. Raising head and shoulders from a prone position occurs by 12 weeks of age, as does looking at the hands while holding them in front of him.

Children who are put to sleep with a bottle of juice or milk are predisposed to the development of otitis media. Normal drainage from the eustachian tube is blocked by the pooling of liquid in the child's mouth.

## QUESTIONS 63-65

The incidence of children ingesting poisonous substances requires teaching parents measures to keep household cleaning agents and medications out of the reach of toddlers and preschool children.

Aspirin is the poison most frequently ingested by children. The immediate treatment is to remove the drug from the child's stomach by inducing vomiting or by gastric lavage.

Hyperventilation is a symptom of salicylate poisoning that causes loss of carbon dioxide and respiratory alkalosis. Other symptoms include increased metabolism, hyperpyrexia, confusion, and loss of consciousness.

Treatment may include the administration of vitamin K to decrease the bleeding tendency.

## QUESTIONS 66-70

Physiologic characteristics of premature infants contribute to the development of physiologic anemia. The diagnosis is confirmed by obtaining hemoglobin and hematocrit determinations.

Nose drops should be administered before feedings. Children naturally breathe through the nose, and nose drops will clear nasal congestion to enable feedings.

When a middle ear infection does not respond to conservative management, a myringotomy is performed to promote drainage from the ear.

For a child who refuses solid food and prefers liquids, a measure that will promote the child's nutrition is withholding liquids until small amounts of solid food are eaten.

## QUESTIONS 71-73

An inguinal hernia usually becomes apparent when the infant is 2 to 3 months of age. The treatment is surgery to prevent incarceration.

Large amounts of the fat-soluble vitamins A and D may be toxic. An overdose of nicotinic acid (Niacin) may also be harmful.

Intramuscular injections for children who are 3 months old should be given into the vastus lateralis muscle.

## QUESTIONS 74-76

A child with laryngotracheobronchitis is placed in a mist tent primarily to increase oxygen and carbon dioxide exchange. Hospitalization is required when respiratory stridor cannot be relieved, hypoxia is present, and temperature is elevated. A tracheostomy may be necessary.

The nursing management of a child with laryngotracheobronchitis requires close observation for signs of respiratory distress. Vital signs are monitored. The child should be permitted to rest as much as possible to conserve his energy. Early signs of hypoxia will be detected by increasing restlessness. Most children respond quickly to treatment but many are prone to recurrence of the condition until they are about 3 years old.

## QUESTIONS 77-80

Early after birth an infant with pyloric stenosis begins to regurgitate or occasionally vomits. As the obstruction in the pylorus continues, the vomiting becomes projectile.

The infant fails to gain and dehydration develops.

Atropine sulfate may cause facial flushing. The action and side effects of atropine should be reviewed. Following surgery, the infant begins to eat, and the weight gain is the best indication that the desired effects have been achieved.

## QUESTIONS 81-84

When a child who is suspected of having an acute appendicitis is admitted, it is important to keep the child on nothing by mouth and determine when the child ate last. If the diagnosis is confirmed, the surgery will be performed without delay as an emergency measure.

The abdominal pain may be generalized or periumbilical, but gradually the most intense pain develops in the right lower quadrant. The child will assume a side-lying position or may be comfortable in a semireclining position.

Diagnostic tests include a complete blood count. An elevated leukocyte count after a history and examination of the child leads to the diagnosis of appendicitis.

Responses to questions by 7 year-olds should be simple, accurate statements.

Barbiturate overdose will cause respiratory depression and may lead to coma and death. Maintaining the patency of the airway always has priority. The level of consciousness will be assessed at regular intervals. An indwelling urethral catheter is inserted to assess kidney function, and urine specimens will be sent to the laboratory for analysis. Intravenous therapy will also be initiated.

Response to treatment will best be indicated by an increasing level of consciousness. When the adolescent becomes alert, the greatest need is to have contact with a sympathetic, supportive person. Being readily available to listen is most important. This is the time to begin preparing the adolescent for the long-term rehabilitation that will be required to overcome the original need to take a drug.

## QUESTIONS 88-92

Injuries occuring out of doors where tetanus spores may be in the soil require investigation of the date of the last tetanus toxoid or tetanus antitoxin administration. Other questions may be asked, but they will have no relevance to the early treatment plan.

Skeletal traction is used primarily to align the ends of the fracture. Immobilization will also prevent further trauma to tissue and will reduce pain.

Whenever a head injury involves a fracture of the skull, careful assessment should be made for evidence of leaking spinal fluid. Headache, edema, and ecchymosis at the site of impact can be expected to occur.

Once the patient's condition is stable, definitive treatment of the fractured extremity is scheduled. Following the application of the long leg cast, it is most important to check pedal pulses. Circulatory impairment in the extremity requires immediate attention.

Discharge teaching for a patient going home with a cast requires detailed instruction in cast care. Keeping the cast intact and keeping it dry are important in the healing of the fracture. Damage to the cast should be reported. The edges of the cast should be covered before discharge to prevent crumbling.

## INDIVIDUAL QUESTIONS 93-100

93. To provide adequate care during the hospitalization of a child who is mentally retarded, it is most important to ask the parents about the child's abilities. Other measures should be carried out for all children admitted to the hospital.

94. A positive response to a tuberculin test indicates that the individual has been infected with the tubercle bacillus. Further diagnostic tests are required to determine the status of the infectious process.

95. The initial feeding of a newborn will reveal the presence of an esophageal atresia with a tracheoesophageal fistula. The infant will begin to choke, since the normal route for swallowing is not present. The abnormality will also cause excessive drooling by the infant.

96. The incidence of battered children makes it essential for health care givers to be alert to evidence of abuse. The behavior of battered children differs from that of children who are well nurtured. When a measure such as a venipuncture is performed, the child will lie still, sense hopelessness, and cry very little, if at all.

97. A parent who abuses a child has difficulty showing concern for the child. The parent usually blames the child for being ill or injured. The parent often has little knowledge of the developmental level that can be expected at a given age and expects the child to function at a higher level. A significant clue to abuse occurs when the parent continually criticizes the child in the presence of other persons.

98. Hemophilia is a bleeding disorder in which there is an absence of an essential factor to clot blood. The disease is transmitted by means of a sex-linked recessive trait. Prolonged bleeding may occur as a result of minor injury.

Treatment includes measures to control the bleeding and to replace deficient factors in the blood. Measures to control bleeding include applying pressure to the area, applying cold compresses, elevating the part, and immobilization of the area. Increased discomfort is an indication that the bleeding is increasing.

99. Children develop gingival hypertrophy as a side effect of Dilantin therapy. Despite meticulous oral hygiene, many children will require a gingivectomy.

100. Following the onset of menarche, menstrual periods may be irregular. The irregularity may be in the timing, the length of the period, or the amount of menstrual flow.

# References for Nursing Care of Children

Gilman, Alfred Goodman, et al. The Pharmacological Basis of Therapeutics, 6th ed. New York: Macmillan Publishing Co., 1980.

Krause, Marie V. and Kathleen Mahan. Food, Nutrition, and Diet Therapy, 7th ed. Philadelphia: W. B. Saunders Co., 1984.

Mott, Sandra R., et al. Nursing Care of Children and Families. Menlo Park, CA: Addison-Wesley Publishing Co., 1985.

Pillitteri, Adele. Child Health Nursing, 2nd ed. Boston: Little, Brown & Co., 1981.

Rodman, Morton J. and Dorothy W. Smith. Pharmacology and Drug Therapy in Nursing, 2nd ed. Philadelphia: J. B. Lippincott Co., 1979.

Scipien, Gladys M., et al. Comprehensive Pediatric Nursing, 2nd ed. New York: McGraw-Hill Book Co., 1979.

Tackett, Jo Joyce Marie, and Mabel Hunsberger. Family-Centered Care of Children and Adolescents, 2nd ed. Philadelphia: W. B. Saunders Co., 1981.

Waechter, Eugenia H., et al. Nursing Care of Children, 10th ed. Philadelphia: J. B. Lippincott Co., 1985.

Whaley, Lucille F. and Donna Wong. Nursing Care of Infants and Children, 2nd ed. St. Louis, MO: The C. V. Mosby Co., 1983.

# PSYCHIATRIC NURSING

Directions: Read each study question carefully. Select one answer from the four choices presented that you think answers the question correctly. There is only one correct answer to each question. Use the answer key to find out whether the answer you selected is the correct one. Read carefully the explanations for the patient situations presented in the study questions, paying particular attention to the explanations for any questions you missed.

---
Mrs. Carol Potter, 43 years old, is admitted to the hospital because of recent overactive behavior. She is too busy to eat or sleep and is losing weight. Mrs. Potter has a history of previous hospitalizations for the same condition. On admission, Mrs. Potter is talking incessantly and her speech is witty, sarcastic, and covers a multitude of topics.
---

1. On admission, Mrs. Potter's care plan should emphasize which of these measures?

   A. Allowing her choices about activities.

   B. Keeping her under constant observation.

   C. Minimizing stimuli in her environment.

   D. Encouraging her to interact with other patients.

2. During Mrs. Potter's early hospitalization, her nursing care plan should provide for which of these needs?

   A. Reality orientation.

   B. Planned rest periods.

   C. Assertiveness training.

   D. Vigorous physical activity.

3. Mrs. Potter enters the dining room for lunch after everyone else is seated and eating. She dashes about telling everyone that she has just been invited to speak at an important meeting of bankers. She then sits down and begins to eat. After taking a few bites, she gets up and walks quickly out of the dining room. To meet Mrs. Potter's nutritional needs, the nurse should take which of these actions initially?

   A. Serve Mrs. Potter her meals in her room.

   B. Give Mrs. Potter finger foods to eat while she is moving around.

   C. Arrange to sit with Mrs. Potter while she has her meals.

   D. Discuss with Mrs. Potter the importance of eating a balanced diet.

4. One day Mrs. Potter is in the dayroom with several other patients. She begins to outline plans for organizing a political rally. No one in the dayroom pays attention to Mrs. Potter, and she becomes frustrated. The nurse should expect that the frustration is most likely to cause Mrs. Potter to exhibit which of these behaviors?

   A. Becoming hostile.

   B. Admitting defeat.

   C. Secluding herself in her room.

   D. Seeking consolation from a staff member.

5. Mrs. Potter is to take lithium carbonate. The nurse should observe her for which of these side effects?

   A. Cardiac arrhythmias.

   B. Lactation.

   C. Glycosuria.

   D. Erythema nodosum.

6. Immediate nursing care plans for Mrs. Potter should serve which of these purposes for her?

   A. To redirect her attention from problems to goals.

   B. To give her recognition.

   C. To reduce her excitement.

   D. To engage her in activities with others.

7. Mrs. Potter's overactive behavior is most probably related to which of these underlying causes?

   A. She finds her life-style boring and inhibiting.

   B. She is warding off depression.

   C. She is unable to manage complex situations.

   D. She has not mastered abstract thinking.

140

Mr. Albert Gorton, 28 years old, is admitted to a psychiatric hospital after expressing suicidal intentions. He has become severely depressed. Five months ago his wife was killed in an automobile accident. Mr. Gorton and his two children have been living with his mother.

8. While Mr. Gorton is severely depressed, which of these measures will be most important?

    A. Providing a cheerful environment for him.

    B. Encouraging him to participate in sports activities.

    C. Giving him a sense of being cared for.

    D. Encouraging him to talk about his wife's death.

9. Mr. Gorton sits in the dayroom for long periods without showing interest in the activities of other patients. He does not answer when spoken to. To help Mr. Gorton at this time, the nurse should take which of these actions?

    A. Encourage him to talk about his children.

    B. Start playing a game in which he may participate.

    C. Give him a humorous short story to read.

    D. Speak to him briefly from time to time without expecting an answer.

10. Tricyclic antidepressant drug therapy is prescribed for Mr. Gorton. The effects of this therapy should begin to occur how long after the therapy is started?

    A. 1 day.

    B. 3 days.

    C. 7 days.

    D. 14 days.

11. Mr. Gorton begins to initiate conversations and his activity increases. He joins a patient group planning a party and agrees to take part in decorating the room to be used. When the time comes to decorate, he is hesitant and expresses his uncertainty about carrying out the task. The nurse should take which of these actions?

    A. Direct Mr. Gorton to talk with the patient committee planning the party.

    B. Encourage Mr. Gorton to proceed with the decorating while arranging for assistance if needed.

    C. Tell Mr. Gorton how disappointed the patients will be if the room is not decorated for the party.

    D. Explore with Mr. Gorton the reason for his reluctance to assume responsibility at this time.

12. Mr. Gorton plays baseball with a group of patients for the first time. When he drops the ball, a patient near him shouts angrily, "Clumsy!" Mr. Gorton leaves the game and sits beside the nurse without making any comment. To ease Mr. Gorton's emotional pain, the nurse should make which of these comments first?

    A. "You're feeling hurt."

    B. "You'll feel better if you stay in the game until it is finished."

    C. "You shouldn't feel bad about making an error in a game that is played for fun."

    D. "Staying in the game would show that you have good team spirit."

Mrs. Agnes Cromwell, 44 years old, is seen in the clinic for depression. Imipramine hydrochloride (Tofranil) is prescribed for her. Mrs. Cromwell fails to keep her clinic appointments, and three months later she is admitted to the psychiatric unit of the hospital. Her husband states that since a prominent person at a social event asked her if he (her husband) was her son, she has spent most of her time in bed. She often did not respond when spoken to and she refused most of the food offered to her. She had stopped taking the prescribed medication because it made her lightheaded. Tofranil is again prescribed.

13. During the acute phase of Mrs. Cromwell's illness, which of these measures should have priority in her care?

A. Keeping her in seclusion.

B. Repeating unit routines to her in detail.

C. Urging her social interaction with other patients.

D. Providing her with physical care.

14. To encourage Mrs. Cromwell to take her medication, the nurse should use which of these approaches?

A. Assure her that the benefits of the drug outweigh the side effects of the drug.

B. Listen to the concerns she expresses about the side effects of the drug.

C. Inform her that medication will be used to control the side effects.

D. Explain to her that the side effects will decrease as her condition improves.

15. The nursing diagnosis for Mrs. Cromwell will most probably indicate that her depression is related to

A. abuse as a child.

B. fear of authority figures.

C. loss of youth.

D. lack of motivation to learn.

16. Mrs. Cromwell arrives at breakfast each morning without having completed her personal grooming. The nurse should take which of these actions?

A. Escort Mrs. Cromwell to her room and supervise her grooming.

B. Explain to Mrs. Cromwell how her grooming needs to be improved.

C. Show Mrs. Cromwell how her grooming differs from that of other patients.

D. Comment favorably on the grooming Mrs. Cromwell has completed.

17. Mrs. Cromwell does not touch the food served to her, but she takes food left by other patients. The nurse should make which of these interpretations of Mrs. Cromwell's behavior?

A. She has a feeling of worthlessness.

B. She is uncomfortable eating with others.

C. She perceives the leaving of food as wasteful.

D. She needs evidence that the food is safe to eat.

18. Mrs. Cromwell begins to improve. Which of these behaviors may be indicative of an impending suicide attempt?

A. Responding sarcastically when asked about her family.

B. Avoiding conversation with some patients on the unit.

C. Identifying with problems expressed by other patients.

D. Appearing detached when walking about the unit.

Mr. Arnold Karton, 20 years old, is admitted to a psychiatric hospital. Mr. Karton has been attending a local college and living at home. His scholastic record has been good. Two months ago he began to eat and sleep poorly and became mute for extended periods of time. He remained in his room and was observed by his parents to grin and point at objects. A diagnosis of schizophrenic reaction is made.

19. When Mr. Karton is admitted to the psychiatric unit, the nurse should take which of these actions first?

A. Escort Mr. Karton to his room.

B. Ask Mr. Karton if he knows where he is.

C. Assure Mr. Karton that he will be well cared for.

D. Introduce Mr. Karton to a few patients.

20. During the first few days of Mr. Karton's hospitalization, which of these measures should have priority?

A. Helping him identify his strengths and weaknesses.

B. Providing him with activities with other patients for short periods.

C. Spending a specified time with him at scheduled intervals.

D. Involving him in setting goals of treatment.

Chlorpromazine hydrochloride (Thorazine) is prescribed for Mr. Karton. For three days, the Thorazine is to be administered intramuscularly.

21. Before administering Thorazine intramuscularly to Mr. Karton, the nurse should make which of these assessments?

A. Checking Mr. Karton's blood pressure.

B. Testing Mr. Karton's urine for the presence of glucose.

C. Testing Mr. Karton's patellar reflexes.

D. Checking laboratory results for Mr. Karton's serum potassium level.

22. While Mr. Karton is taking Thorazine, he should be observed for which of these symptoms?

A. Pseudoparkinsonism.

B. Dehydration.

C. Manic excitement.

D. Urinary retention.

Mrs. Mary Carter, a 32-year-old divorced mother, comes to the mental health center. The family has had repeated crises, and Mrs. Carter complains of being overwhelmed. She has a 12-year-old son who is often truant from school, a 10-year-old daughter who has asthma, a 7-year-old daughter who has learning disabilities, and a 6-year-old son. The children's father, who is employed, has been delinquent in his child-support payments for several weeks.

23. When considering a plan to assist Mrs. Carter with her crisis situation, which of these approaches will be most important initially?

A. Determining the methods Mrs. Carter uses to solve problems.

B. Conveying to Mrs. Carter that she is a competent person.

C. Exploring the availability of community agencies that may assist Mrs. Carter.

D. Helping Mrs. Carter to minimize the gravity of her situation.

24. The nurse suggests that Mrs. Carter contact an attorney about obtaining child-support payments from her ex-husband and that she talk with the school psychologist about her son's truancy. The nurse's approach is intended primarily to achieve which of these goals?

A. To relieve Mrs. Carter of some of her responsibilities.

B. To support Mrs. Carter's ability to solve problems.

C. To demonstrate to Mrs. Carter how to set priorities.

D. To establish a support system for Mrs. Carter.

25. The next day, Mrs. Carter returns to the clinic and says that she was unable to get appointments for that day with the attorney or the school psychologist. She expresses the feeling that the urgency of her problems was not recognized. To help Mrs. Carter at this time, which of these interventions would be most important?

A. Telephone for the appointments Mrs. Carter is seeking to make.

B. Explore with Mrs. Carter alternate solutions to her problems.

C. Support Mrs. Carter in developing perseverence in her efforts.

D. Explain to Mrs. Carter how her panic intensifies the seriousness of her situation.

---

Mr. Ralph Bond, a 58-year-old supervisor who is married, is admitted to the psychiatric hospital. Mr. Bond expected a job promotion two months ago, but a younger employee was promoted to the position instead. Mr. Bond became upset and increasingly suspicious. He began to accuse his wife of being unfaithful and uncaring although he had no evidence. After the family physician recommended psychiatric therapy, Mr. Bond was outraged. He began threatening his wife, and when he did attack her, the police were summoned, and Mr. Bond was brought to the hospital.

---

26. Mr. Bond's history indicates that his recent behavior is basically related to which of these problems?

A. Premature senility.

B. Lack of role identification.

C. Economic insecurity.

D. Poor self-esteem.

27. Mr. Bond expresses anger and the belief that his wife called the police because she wanted him to leave their home. Initiating a therapeutic relationship with Mr. Bond while he is acutely ill will probably require which of these measures by the nurse?

A. Explaining to Mr. Bond the basis of his delusions.

B. Telling Mr. Bond how the nurse plans to get to know him.

C. Considering Mr. Bond's need to remain emotionally distant.

D. Questioning Mr. Bond about his suspiciousness.

28. Mr. Bond's plan of care should focus on which of these areas initially?

A. His need for a promotion.

B. His relationship with his wife.

C. His ability to verbalize feelings in a direct way.

D. His self-control.

29. A young man who is a patient walks by Mr. Bond's room while Mr. Bond is standing in the doorway talking to the nurse. Mr. Bond says, "He's here to get rid of me." To clarify Mr. Bond's statement, the nurse should ask him which of these questions?

A. "When did you first notice that man?"

B. "Have you had a conversation with that man?"

C. "Do you recognize something about that man that bothers you?"

D. "Does that man live in your neighborhood?"

30. Mr. Bond walks toward the nurse's desk and observes the nurse making a telephone call. A few minutes later, Mr. Bond accuses the nurse of having called the police. The nurse should interpret Mr. Bond's behavior as

A. projection.

B. reaction formation.

C. transference.

D. ideas of reference.

31. To facilitate communication with a suspicious patient such as Mr. Bond, the nurse should

A. ask him direct questions.

B. use concrete words.

C. indicate agreement even when his meaning is unclear.

D. offer evidence to disprove his false beliefs.

-------------------------------------------------
Miss Laura Landry, 36 years old, is admitted to the psychiatric unit of the hospital after extensive diagnostic tests established no physical basis for her persistent complaints of headache, fatigue, and difficulty in swallowing.
-------------------------------------------------

32. During the first interview with Miss Landry, which of these assessments would be needed immediately to plan her nursing care?

A. What is her level of anxiety?

B. When did she begin having these symptoms?

C. Does she have significant others?

D. What does she say to herself when under stress?

33. When Miss Landry does not appear for the evening meal, the nurse goes to Miss Landry's room. Miss Landry is lying on the bed, crying, and stating that she is physically ill. The nurse should take which of these actions?

A. Tell Miss Landry that she will feel better after she eats.

B. Escort Miss Landry to the dining room.

C. Inform Miss Landry that her meal will be served to her in her room.

D. Talk with Miss Landry before deciding about plans for her meal.

34. After the nurse has had several brief conversations with Miss Landry, Miss Landry suddenly says, "I'm afraid to ride in an elevator. I know it's silly, but I can't help it." Which of these responses by the nurse would be the best example of acknowledgement?

A. "It's hard to manage without using elevators."

B. "Being afraid to ride in elevators seems unreasonable to you."

C. "Perhaps you should consider why you are afraid to ride in an elevator."

D. "The speed of elevators frightens you."

35. One day, Miss Landry says to the nurse, "The doctor doesn't believe me when I say I am sick. He doesn't know that tests don't show everything." The nurse should use which of these approaches in responding to Miss Landry?

A. Show acceptance of Miss Landry's opinion.

B. Explain to Miss Landry that her complaints are not symptoms of a specific illness.

C. Ask Miss Landry to repeat her conversation with the physician.

D. Inform Miss Landry that an error in diagnostic test results is unlikely.

36. During the next two weeks, Miss Landry has several conferences with the psychiatrist. She becomes increasingly anxious, and her physical symptoms intensify. The nurse should make which of these interpretations of these observations?

A. Miss Landry needs to be involved in modifying the goals of therapy.

B. Miss Landry may be developing a physical illness unrelated to her emotional problems.

C. Miss Landry is responding to therapy as expected at this time.

D. Miss Landry is probably beginning to have insight into her behavior.

----

David Baxton, 22 months old, may be autistic. His mother brings him to the child mental health clinic.

----

37. During an interview with the nurse, Mrs. Baxton makes all of the following statements about David's behavior until he was one year old. Which statement most strongly suggests that David may be autistic?

A. "He was a good baby and rarely cried when I left the room."

B. "He slept very well after each feeding."

C. "He spit out every new food the first time I gave it to him."

D. "He started to walk without learning to crawl first."

38. In attempting to establish a therapeutic relationship with David, the nurse should expect to encounter which of these problems?

A. Hallucinating.

B. Impaired hearing.

C. Bizarre behavior.

D. Clinging to others.

39. To initiate a relationship with a child such as David, who may be autistic, the nurse would probably be most effective by using which of these approaches?

A. Playing peek-a-boo.

B. Having him point to designated body parts.

C. Sitting with him.

D. Telling him a story.

----

Mrs. Anna Krell, 49 years old, is admitted to the detoxification unit. She admits to drinking increasingly larger amounts of alcohol for the past 5 years. Mrs. Krell's husband accompanies her, and he states that he has threatened to leave her unless she has treatment. Mrs. Krell states that she had her last drink one hour ago.

----

40. The morning after admission, Mrs. Krell is restless, tremulous, and somewhat agitated. The nurse should take which of these actions at this time?

A. Obtain an order for lithium carbonate for Mrs. Krell.

B. Observe Mrs. Krell's behavior closely.

C. Darken Mrs. Krell's room.

D. Prepare to place Mrs. Krell in restraints.

41. Mrs. Krell should be observed for the development of which of these objective symptoms?

A. Hypersomnia.

B. Pilomotor erection (gooseflesh).

C. Convulsions.

D. Dermatitis.

146

42. Two nights later, Mrs. Krell runs out of her room. She is confused and disoriented. She says, "Let me out of here. Bugs are crawling all over that room." The nurse should take which of these actions?

A. Escort Mrs. Krell back to her room and show her that there is nothing to fear.

B. Assist Mrs. Krell back into bed and then search her room for alcohol.

C. Take Mrs. Krell to a quiet area and ask her if she has had nightmares in the past.

D. Have a staff member stay with Mrs. Krell and notify the physician.

------------------------------------------------
Mrs. Krell develops delirium tremens.
------------------------------------------------

43. At this time, which of these nursing diagnoses should be given priority in caring for Mrs. Krell?

A. Potential for physical injury related to impulsiveness.

B. Noncompliance with medical regimen related to denial of illness.

C. Anticipatory grieving related to her husband's threat of abandoning her.

D. Translocation syndrome related to transfer to a strange environment.

44. Which of these goals will be most important while Mrs. Krell has delirium tremens?

A. To increase her ability to cope with stresses.

B. To maintain the support of significant others.

C. To support her physical adaptation.

D. To acknowledge that she is dependent on alcohol.

------------------------------------------------
Mrs. Krell recovers from delirium tremens. She agrees to participate in group therapy sessions for a period before being discharged.
------------------------------------------------

45. Initially, group therapy may have which of these effects on Mrs. Krell?

A. She will develop insight into her reasons for needing alcohol.

B. She will experience periods of extreme anxiety.

C. She will be able to set realistic goals for herself.

D. She will be able to identify the personality traits she needs to change.

46. Mrs. Krell is to receive disulfiram (Antabuse). The medication is prescribed for which of these purposes?

A. To minimize the effects of alcohol.

B. To improve detoxification by the liver.

C. To increase her utilization of vitamins.

D. To help her refrain from drinking alcohol.

47. Mrs. Krell asks the nurse about participation in Alcoholics Anonymous. In addition to arranging for a visit by a worker from Alcoholics Anonymous, the nurse should explain that the primary purpose of the organization is to

A. explore the individual member's need for dependence on alcohol.

B. help members maintain abstinence from alcohol.

C. teach members how to manage social situations without the need for alcohol.

D. increase public awareness of the results of alcoholism.

48. Before Mrs. Krell is discharged, it is important that she have which of these understandings about a rehabilitation program for alcoholics?

A. It is a long-term therapy.

B. It requires family participation to be successful.

C. It will necessitate restructuring social situations.

D. It fosters intolerance of substance abusers.

---

Mr. Donald Sommer, 22 years old, has a long history of truancy and delinquency. He has been addicted to heroin for four years. His employer has threatened to fire him because of frequent absenteeism. Mr. Sommer agrees to be admitted to a drug detoxification unit for treatment. A diagnosis of antisocial personality disorder is made.

---

49. Which of these comments, if made by Mr. Sommer, would demonstrate an expected attitude about unit rules and regulations?

A. "Rules and regulations do not apply to me."

B. "I am accused of breaking rules and regulations when I am really following them."

C. "I know rules and regulations are for my benefit."

D. "Rules and regulations get changed when I do something somebody doesn't like."

50. Mr. Sommer tells the physician that he cannot talk with the nurses, and then he tells the nurses that he cannot talk with the physician. Since Mr. Sommer plays one staff member against another, it will be important to take which of these measures?

A. Planning a conference with staff involved with Mr. Sommer's care to deal with the problem.

B. Informing staff members when Mr. Sommer makes comments that criticize them.

C. Ignoring Mr. Sommer's statements about the staff.

D. Interpreting Mr. Sommer's remarks about staff as reflecting insight into his own lack of trust in people.

---

Mrs. Glenda Hardy, 35 years old, is accompanied by her husband when she is admitted to the psychiatric hospital. Mr. Hardy reports that his wife has been crying for about two weeks and any effort at communicating with her causes another flood of tears. She has eaten very little and refuses efforts by her husband to spoon-feed her. Mrs. Hardy occasionally shakes her head and says, "I'm no good. I should die." Mrs. Hardy was employed as a secretary until a month ago, when the company she worked for moved to another state.

---

51. Since Mrs. Hardy has not been eating, which of these approaches should be used to provide her with nourishment at this time?

A. Giving her finger foods to eat.

B. Allowing her to select foods she likes.

C. Indicating to her that she is expected to eat the foods provided.

D. Keeping liquid diet supplements in her room.

52. Mrs. Hardy tells the nurse that she is useless and that she should not live any longer. Which of these responses should the nurse make?

A. Acknowledge Mrs. Hardy's statements.

B. Remind Mrs. Hardy of her husband's concern for her.

C. Ask Mrs. Hardy what efforts she made to get another secretarial job.

D. Encourage Mrs. Hardy to be specific about her deficiencies.

53. Amitriptyline hydrochloride (Elavil) is prescribed for Mrs. Hardy. After taking the drug for ten days, Mrs. Hardy tells the nurse that the drug is not helping her. Which of these judgments should the nurse make about Mrs. Hardy's comment?

A. Mrs. Hardy needs larger doses of Elavil.

B. Mrs. Hardy does not recognize the changes that Elavil has made in her behavior.

C. Mrs. Hardy has not been taking Elavil long enough for it to have become effective.

D. Mrs. Hardy may be resistant to Elavil.

54. Mrs. Hardy agrees to go on an outing with a group of patients. She is sitting waiting for the group to gather. The nurse observes that Mrs. Hardy's clothing is soiled and that she has not combed her hair. The nurse should take which of these actions?

A. Allow Mrs. Hardy to go as she is.

B. Ask Mrs. Hardy why she did not dress for the occasion.

C. Help Mrs. Hardy with her grooming.

D. Ask the other patients to comment on Mrs. Hardy's appearance.

---------------------------------------------------
Miss Carol Franey, 24 years old, is being seen in the clinic for numerous physical complaints. The results of diagnostic tests reveal no physical defect, and it is determined that her complaints are due to anxiety.
---------------------------------------------------

55. When planning care for Miss Franey, it would be most important to include which of these understandings about her behavior?

A. She is not reliable when giving information.

B. She is deliberately avoiding responsibilities.

C. She is demanding primary gains.

D. She is experiencing the discomfort she reports.

56. Miss Franey's care plan should include which of these measures?

A. Providing opportunities for her to discuss her reasons for avoiding responsibility.

B. Arranging time for her to express her concerns.

C. Encouraging her to seek diversional interests.

D. Explaining to her the emotional basis for her physical complaints.

57. While Miss Franey is experiencing severe anxiety, the nurse would be most supportive by using which of these approaches?

A. Indicating to Miss Franey an understanding of her perceptions of her situation.

B. Discussing with Miss Franey alternative solutions to her problems.

C. Assessing Miss Franey's physical complaints at regular intervals.

D. Pointing out to Miss Franey the inadequacy of her defenses.

58. Miss Franey explains her physical symptoms at great length. The nurse should plan to take which of these actions?

A. Ask Miss Franey for specific details about her symptoms.

B. Agree with Miss Franey's statements about her symptoms.

C. Remind Miss Franey that there is no physical basis for her symptoms.

D. Attempt to reward Miss Franey when she is not discussing her symptoms.

----------------------------------------
Mrs. Doris Miller, 86 years old, is admitted to the psychiatric unit of an extended care facility. She has become very confused and was found wandering about her neighborhood without knowing where she lived.
----------------------------------------

59. Mrs. Miller has diminished sensory perception. The nurse should therefore expect Mrs. Miller to demonstrate which of these behaviors?

A. She will have complaints of pain unrelated to her physical condition.

B. She will dress too warmly or too lightly for the temperature of her environment.

C. She will anger other patients by her insensitivity in social situations.

D. She will ask the same question repeatedly in an effort to gain acceptance from those around her.

60. When directed to get dressed in the morning, Mrs. Miller sits with a garment in her hands, unable to proceed. The nurse should take which of these actions?

A. Identify each article of clothing as the nurse puts it on Mrs. Miller.

B. Give Mrs. Miller step-by-step directions for putting her clothing on.

C. Give Mrs. Miller a time limit in which to put on her clothing.

D. Remind Mrs. Miller that she must be dressed in order to be permitted to carry out the activities for the day.

61. To provide Mrs. Miller with the greatest sense of well-being, her care plan should include which of these measures?

A. Emphasizing diversity and surprise in the daily activities.

B. Scheduling major activities at the same time each day.

C. Maintaining sameness in all aspects of the daily routine.

D. Having Mrs. Miller plan her schedule each morning.

62. Maximum emotional support will be provided for Mrs. Miller by which of these measures?

A. Encouraging Mrs. Miller to talk about the past.

B. Providing assistance before Mrs. Miller shows need of it.

C. Having Mrs. Miller demonstrate recall of recent events.

D. Planning time for Mrs. Miller to complete activities at her own pace.

63. Mrs. Miller begins to take bread from each meal and hide it among her belongings. To discourage this behavior, the nurse should take which of these approaches?

A. Explain to Mrs. Miller that food will attract insects.

B. Remind Mrs. Miller that food is provided at least three times a day.

C. Give Mrs. Miller a secure container for the food.

D. Have Mrs. Miller give up her hoard after each meal.

Mr. Paul Trumbull, 41 years old, is admitted to the psychiatric unit for treatment of anxiety neurosis. For several weeks, Mr. Trumbull has had increasingly frequent periods of palpitations, sweating, chest pain, and choking.

----------------------------------------

64. Mr. Trumbull's nursing diagnosis is "severe anxiety, stressor unidentified." Which of these measures is appropriate during Mr. Trumbull's attacks?

A. Supporting and protecting him.

B. Engaging him in socially productive behavior.

C. Having him review the circumstances that precipitated the symptoms.

D. Ignoring him until the symptoms subside.


65. To master his anxiety, Mr. Trumbull must first

A. recognize that he is feeling anxious.

B. identify the situations that precipitated his anxiety.

C. understand the basis for his anxiety.

D. select a strategy to cope with his anxiety.

Miss Emily Durby, 46 years old, has been hospitalized since she was a young adult. She is mute and spends most of the day sitting on the floor with her head resting on her knees. She will occasionally get up quickly, dash around the room, and then reposition herself on the floor. Her care includes having a nurse spend an hour with her during the day and another hour during the evening.

----------------------------------------

66. The nurse should understand that mutism for Miss Durby probably serves which of these purposes?

A. To punish herself.

B. To attract attention.

C. To deny mental deterioration.

D. To protect herself.


67. Which of these measures in Miss Durby's care plan should be most important?

A. Encouraging her to have an adequate intake of fluids.

B. Scheduling periods of active exercise for her.

C. Monitoring her physical condition.

D. Maintaining her personal hygiene.


68. One evening while the nurse is sitting next to Miss Durby, Miss Durby suddenly begins to say something, but it is incoherent. The nurse should make which of these responses?

A. "I would like to understand what you are saying, Miss Durby."

B. "You are not speaking clearly, Miss Durby."

C. "It's nice to hear you making a sound, Miss Durby."

D. "I have never heard you speak before, Miss Durby."

69. Miss Durby begins to verbalize more frequently. One day she tells the nurse that parts of her body do not seem to belong to her. Considering Miss Durby's difficulty with body boundaries, her nursing orders should include which of these directions?

A. Touch her frequently to stimulate her touch receptors.

B. Warn her before touching her to prevent panic.

C. Engage her in pantomime to enhance her self-awareness.

D. Have her practice meditation to reduce her anxiety.

70. Several months later, one of the nurses who spends time with Miss Durby is absent from work for a week due to illness. When the nurse returns and greets Miss Durby, Miss Durby says, "You left me like all the rest. I was all alone again." To reestablish a therapeutic relationship, the nurse should make which of these responses?

A. "I had to leave you, Miss Durby. I was ill."

B. "You were not alone, Miss Durby. Another nurse spent time with you."

C. "It's all right to be upset when I had to be away. You thought I wasn't interested in you."

D. "I'm glad you missed me. Now I know you like me."

---

Mr. Thomas Randolph, 19 years old, is admitted to the hospital with an antisocial personality disorder. He has a history of delinquent acts, such as breaking into the homes of family friends and raiding their refrigerator or taking their sports equipment without permission. Most recently, he entered the garage of family friends and drove away with their car. He has considerable charm and presents reasons for his behavior that he perceives as rational. He fails to see any defect in his behavior.

---

71. Since Mr. Randolph controls his anxiety through socially aggressive patterns, it is most important to include which of these measures in his care?

A. Planning activities for Mr. Randolph that he selects.

B. Maintaining set limits on Mr. Randolph's behavior.

C. Planning levels of activities that Mr. Randolph must achieve before advancing to more independent activities.

D. Promoting Mr. Randolph's self-image by having him direct selected group activities.

72. Mr. Randolph seeks the attention of a young, attractive nurse, and he finds many excuses to involve the nurse in conversation. The nurse should have which of these understandings of this situation?

A. The nurse should help Mr. Randolph.

B. The nurse is responsible for maintaining a therapeutic relationship with Mr. Randolph.

C. The nurse should prepare to act as an advocate for Mr. Randolph.

D. The nurse is uniquely able to gain Mr. Randolph's confidence.

73. Mr. Randolph begins to behave in all of the following ways. Which behavior indicates an improvement in his condition?

A. He offers a detailed plan for a recreational activity.

B. He expresses his anger directly at a person who frustrated him.

C. He expresses concern about the depressed affect of another patient.

D. He offers logical explanations for his past delinquent behaviors.

74. Mr. Randolph says to the nurse, "I have something to tell you because I know you can keep a secret." To respond to his statement, the nurse should make which of these remarks?

A. "It's nice that you trust me to keep a secret."

B. "I would like to hear your secret."

C. "I cannot promise that I can keep your secret."

D. "A secret is not a secret when it is repeated."

---

Mrs. Freida Winter, 73 years old, has been widowed for ten years. She was forced to vacate her apartment several months ago when fire destroyed the building. Mrs. Winter has been wandering about the city, begging for money to buy food and sleeping on park benches or in secluded areas of large buildings. She carries her personal belongings in three bundles. One day she enters the bus terminal and becomes very noisy and quarrelsome. The police are called, and she is brought to a psychiatric unit.

---

75. To plan care for Mrs. Winter, which of these actions should be taken first?

A. Determine her interests.

B. Obtain information about her family.

C. Identify her emotional needs.

D. Evaluate her physical condition.

76. When Mrs. Winter is admitted, she is asked to keep her possessions in a locker that is in her room. She insists on removing several articles to carry around with her. She constantly drops or misplaces them, and then she accuses people of stealing from her. Which of these plans by the nurse would probably meet Mrs. Winter's needs and minimize problems with other patients?

A. Clean out Mrs. Winter's useless possessions when she is not in her room.

B. Inform Mrs. Winter that her belongings may be lost if she does not keep them stored in her room.

C. Help Mrs. Winter to select a few items that she can easily manage to carry with her while leaving the rest in the storage area.

D. Tell Mrs. Winter that being argumentative over her possessions will make other patients dislike her.

77. Mrs. Winter continues to carry most of her possessions around with her. The nurse should make which of these interpretations of this behavior?

A. Mrs. Winter needs to keep busy.

B. Mrs. Winter needs to maintain her identity.

C. Mrs. Winter needs to be a focus of attention.

D. Mrs. Winter needs a means of becoming involved with others.

78. It is determined that Mrs. Winter should be transferred to a skilled nursing facility. She is interested in this arrangement, but she expresses considerable anxiety about it. To minimize Mrs. Winter's stress relating to the transfer, the nurse should take which of these measures?

A. Point out to Mrs. Winter that the nursing home is probably not so very different from the institution she is in.

B. Assure Mrs. Winter that the transfer is in her best interest.

C. Arrange for Mrs. Winter to visit the nursing home.

D. Describe to Mrs. Winter the facilities that will be available to her.

---

Mrs. Magda Long, 28 years old, is accompanied by her husband when she is admitted to the psychiatric unit. Mrs. Long remains motionless and says nothing. Mr. Long reports that his wife has become withdrawn from social situations, and that most recently she remained secluded in a darkened room and sat for long periods without moving.

---

79. To plan care for Mrs. Long, priority should be given to which of these assessments?

A. What does she do for herself?

B. When did her symptoms begin?

C. Is she a danger to herself or others?

D. Can she be induced to give information about herself?

80. To deal with Mrs. Long's withdrawal, the nurse should begin by first

A. eliciting Mrs. Long's felt needs.

B. observing Mrs. Long's reaction to other patients.

C. remaining with Mrs. Long for scheduled periods.

D. asking Mrs. Long questions she can answer with "yes" or "no."

81. Because Mrs. Long remains immobile for extended periods, it will be essential to include which of these measures in her care?

A. Exercising her extremities.

B. Providing environmental stimuli.

C. Teaching other coping mechanisms.

D. Prompting reality testing.

82. Assuming that Mrs. Long's greatest anxiety results from interpersonal closeness, which of these behaviors would indicate the highest level of response to treatment?

A. She begins to assume responsibility for her personal care.

B. She makes eye contact with the nurse.

C. She says she has to go home.

D. She eats in the dining room with other patients.

---

The remainder of the questions are individual questions.

---

83. A male patient in a psychiatric unit becomes increasingly agitated in spite of attempts by the staff to curb his behavior. The patient begins to overturn furniture in the dayroom and shouts threats to everyone near him. The nurse should take which of these actions first?

A. Obtain enough assistance to control the patient.

B. Orient the patient to person and place.

C. Leave the patient alone in the dayroom until he calms himself.

D. Determine if the patient has an order for a sedative.

84. A nurse on a psychiatric unit is assisting patients to establish a self-government group. To achieve the desired goals, the nurse should take which of these roles in the planning?

A. Providing leadership.

B. Assigning responsibility to each patient.

C. Explaining the desired organizational structure.

D. Setting limits of responsibility.

85. A female patient who is terminally ill says to the nurse, "I'm afraid to die. I wish I could talk to my family about it." To be helpful to the patient, the nurse should make which of these comments?

A. "I will be glad to talk to your family."

B. "I'll call the hospital chaplain to talk with you."

C. "I have heard your feelings expressed by others many times."

D. "I would like to hear more about your concerns."

86. Mrs. Emma Bonner, 51 years old, had a right mastectomy four days ago. Her postoperative recovery has been good. Mrs. Bonner is in a room with three other patients. When the nurse enters the room, all the patients are in bed. As the nurse approaches Mrs. Bonner, Mrs. Bonner is crying quietly, with her head turned toward the wall. Mrs. Bonner states that she wishes to be alone.

The nurse should take which of these actions?

A. Ask the patients in Mrs. Bonner's room if they observed an incident that could have upset Mrs. Bonner.

B. Pull the curtains around Mrs. Bonner's bed before leaving her bedside.

C. Tell Mrs. Bonner that it would be better to talk about whatever is troubling her.

D. Obtain an order for sedation to administer to Mrs. Bonner.

87. A patient is brought to the emergency room after taking an overdose of medication. It would be most important to ask which of these questions first?

A. How much medication was taken?

B. Who prescribed the medication?

C. At what time was the medication taken?

D. What medication was taken?

88. The staff on a unit plan to initiate a remotivation program for several elderly patients who are inactive and preoccupied with themselves. The staff's planning should consider which of these questions first?

A. Are there any similarities in the physical abilities of these patients?

B. What activities would stimulate the senses of these patients?

C. Do these patients have similar interests?

D. Can these patients contribute their ideas?

89. The desired therapeutic effect of patient government will have been achieved when the patients exhibit which of these behaviors?

A. They plan activities as a group.

B. They determine the punishment for violators of unit rules.

C. They discuss grievances in a matter-of-fact manner.

D. They demonstrate an increased sense of responsibility.

90. The nurse approaches a patient who is having auditory hallucinations. The patient says, "Do you hear those people? It's awful what they're saying!" The nurse should respond in which of these ways?

A. "Do you know the people?"

B. "I do not hear people talking."

C. "Tell me what the people are saying."

D. "Are the people angry about something?"

155

91. An elderly patient repeats a story about her parents' great wealth and prominence during her childhood to everyone who speaks to her. Which of these interpretations should be made of this behavior?

A. She is seeking self-esteem.

B. She enjoys recalling the pleasures of her youth.

C. She has lost the ability to remember recent events.

D. She is expressing interest in talking with people.

92. The nurse discusses with a foster mother the care of a child who is mentally retarded. Which of these measures will be most important in the child's care?

A. Following a routine when carrying out the child's daily activities.

B. Using a time-out room for the child.

C. Teaching the child a new activity each week.

D. Observing the child's interaction with other children.

93. When counseling a victim of rape immediately after the incident, which of these goals is most important?

A. To support the victim during the physical examination.

B. To support the victim in filing legal charges.

C. To restore the victim's emotional control.

D. To restore the victim's sense of worth.

94. The treatment goal for a patient with severe anxiety will have been achieved when the patient demonstrates which of these behaviors?

A. The patient recognizes the source of the anxiety.

B. The patient is able to use the anxiety constructively.

C. The patient can function without any sense of anxiety.

D. The patient identifies the physical effects of the anxiety.

95. A 20-year-old male patient has an ileostomy, and his condition is satisfactory. When the nurse changes the ileostomy appliance, the patient turns his head away and closes his eyes. To help the patient deal with the change in his body image, which of these comments should the nurse make initially?

A. "Your stoma looks good."

B. "You'll feel better once you look at the stoma."

C. "I will begin to teach you to take care of the stoma."

D. "It's difficult to look at the stoma the first time."

96. A patient who is hospitalized for treatment of an intestinal obstruction has multiple complaints about the hospital services and personnel. To care for the patient, it would be useful for the nurse to have which of these understandings of such behavior?

A. A person reacts to illness in ways that are similar to the person's reactions to other stressful experiences.

B. A person's reaction to hospitalization is determined by the person's previous experiences in a hospital.

C. A person who is hospitalized has to adopt new defenses.

D. A person's reaction to illness and hospitalization is determined by the seriousness of the person's condition.

97. A woman's emotional responses to having a hysterectomy will be influenced most strongly by which of these personal characteristics?

   A. Her social status.

   B. Her education.

   C. Her culture.

   D. Her self-image.


98. When the nurse detects that a patient is using defense mechanisms, the nurse should make which of these interpretations of the patient's behavior?

   A. The patient is attempting to reestablish emotional equilibrium.

   B. The patient is using self-defeating measures.

   C. The patient is demonstrating illness.

   D. The patient is asking for support from significant others.


This is the end of the study questions for Psychiatric Nursing. Check to see whether you selected the correct answer to each question by using the answer key on page 158. Explanations for the correct answers in each patient situation begin on page 159. Read the explanations carefully, paying particular attention to the explanations for any questions you answered incorrectly. Then select a reference book from the list of recommended texts on page 178. Read the section that pertains to each patient situation presented in the study questions.

# Answer Key to Study Questions
## for Psychiatric Nursing

| | | | | |
|---|---|---|---|---|
| 1. C | 21. A | 41. C | 61. B | 81. A |
| 2. B | 22. A | 42. D | 62. D | 82. B |
| 3. B | 23. B | 43. A | 63. C | 83. A |
| 4. A | 24. B | 44. C | 64. A | 84. D |
| 5. A | 25. C | 45. B | 65. A | 85. D |
| 6. C | 26. D | 46. D | 66. D | 86. B |
| 7. B | 27. C | 47. B | 67. C | 87. D |
| 8. C | 28. D | 48. A | 68. A | 88. B |
| 9. D | 29. C | 49. A | 69. B | 89. D |
| 10. D | 30. D | 50. A | 70. C | 90. B |
| 11. B | 31. B | 51. C | 71. B | 91. A |
| 12. A | 32. A | 52. A | 72. B | 92. A |
| 13. D | 33. D | 53. C | 73. C | 93. C |
| 14. B | 34. B | 54. C | 74. C | 94. B |
| 15. C | 25. A | 55. D | 75. D | 95. D |
| 16. D | 36. C | 56. B | 76. C | 96. A |
| 17. A | 37. A | 57. A | 77. B | 97. D |
| 18. D | 38. C | 58. D | 78. C | 98. A |
| 19. A | 39. C | 59. B | 79. C | |
| 20. C | 40. B | 60. B | 80. C | |

# Explanations for Study Questions
# for Psychiatric Nursing

The client is demonstrating the overactive behavior and elated mood of a manic disorder. Review the characteristics of affect, thought, and motor activity of a manic disorder; the underlying psychodynamics; and the defenses used most prominently. Review the cyclical pattern that may involve manic and depressive episodes.

A decreased attention span, heightened distractibility, and inappropriate social judgment must be considered when planning nursing intervention for the manic client. The general activity of the treatment unit is likely to be too stimulating for the client on admission; thus, measures must be taken to reduce stimuli as much as possible. This may require having the client spend at least part of the time in a quiet room in the presence of a staff member.

The client's incessant activity and failure to respond adequately to physiological needs pose potential problems of exhaustion, dehydration, malnutrition, and physical injury. Priority must be given to meeting basic needs, such as planned rest periods.

Since the client may claim to be too busy to eat, nourishment must be provided so that she can eat frequently while moving about.

The client's superficial cheerfulness and expansiveness can quickly turn to anger and hostility when she is thwarted or when she encounters controls and consequently perceives a threat to her self-esteem. Question #4 illustrates this concept.

Since lithium carbonate is the drug of choice in manic or manic-depressive illness, the nurse must be familiar with its action and side effects, as well as the nursing interventions that are indicated for clients receiving this medication. Cardiac arrhythmias may be a side effect of lithium carbonate. Reducing the client's excitement is fundamental to setting other goals of treatment.

The dynamics of manic behavior reveal that the individual is, in fact, using elation and hyperactivity as a defense against depression.

Additional problems that should be considered in the nursing care of a manic client include: meddlesomeness and intru- siveness into the activities of others; manipulativeness; teasing, taunting, and sarcasm. The client's hostility often takes the form of verbal attacks upon the most vulnerable aspects of others--both clients and staff. Because of the socially uninhibited and often sexually provocative behavior of manic clients, it is necessary to establish controls that will protect them from incurring rejection and derision, which will further damage their self-esteem.

In contrast to clients experiencing a schizophrenic reaction, manic clients usually seem in better contact with reality. While their speech may be rapid, with many puns, jokes, and switches from one topic to another (flight of ideas), their verbal communication is usually easier to comprehend than that of the schizophrenic. The nurse should remember, however, that the manic client's rapid flow of conversation is usually on a superficial level and is a prominent example of the client's denial of his or her illness.

## QUESTIONS 8-12

The client's severe depression occurs after the sudden death of his wife. He has not resolved the grief associated with her death.

Review the levels of depression and the accepted diagnostic labels used to distinguish various types of depression. Review the charac-teristics of affect, thought, and behavior in depression; theories explaining the development of depression; and the responses that are commonly elicited by the client's symptoms.

Among the problems that must be addressed in caring for the depressed client is the alleviation of his extremely low self-esteem and sense of hopelessness and helplessness. Initially this requires acceptance of him at his current level of functioning and a demonstration of concern by the nurse, with minimal demands being made upon him for social interaction. An environment or interpersonal approach that suggests cheerfulness will only reinforce his inability to see the possibility of hope or relief at this time.

Since one of the group of drugs known as tricyclic antidepressants is often used in the treatment of depression, the nurse should be familiar with their actions, side effects, and nursing implications.

The depressed client's initial efforts to participate in social activities should be encouraged by the nurse. Care must be taken not to make the client feel guilty if his efforts are not successful. Acknowledge the client's feelings about success or failure in activities; avoid telling him how he should feel. Questions #11 and #12 illustrate the use of this nursing intervention.

## QUESTIONS 13-18

A client who is hospitalized because of depression demonstrates some of the vegetative signs of depression. The slowing down of body movements and somatic activity and the failure to eat or to maintain self-care demand priority in the plan of care.

The client's reluctance to take the prescribed antidepressant medication must be addressed. First she should be encouraged to express her feelings about the side effects that she experienced when she took the drug before hospitalization. This acknowledgement of her concerns precedes any explanation of the value of the drug or how side effects may be alleviated.

The client has a sense of loss of her youth and confrontation with middle age as a result of a prominent person asking if her husband was her son. Question #16 contrasts a positive approach with less therapeutic interventions that emphasize the client's deficits.

The nurse must be alert to behavior by the client that gives evidence of her feelings of worthlessness. Taking the leftovers of other patients is a way of saying: "I deserve only what is cast off by others."

As the depressed client begins to improve, the risk of suicide is increased because the person now has a greater amount of energy. Nursing staff must be extremely observant of any behavioral signs that may indicate that the client is planning a suicide attempt. These behaviors may include a sudden lightening of mood, an air of relaxation, or the appearance of detachment.

## QUESTIONS 19-22

The client's social isolation, disturbances in motor activity, mutism, inappropriate affect, and seemingly meaningless activity are suggestive of a schizophrenic disorder.

Review the biological and psychosocial theories that attempt to explain the development of schizophrenia. Review the disturbances in thinking, affect, and behavior that are characteristic of schizophrenia, and the significant problems that usually must be addressed in the plan of care.

The client who is experiencing an acute schizophrenic disorder may be extremely anxious, suspicious, and fearful of the unfamiliar environment he is entering. The nurse should approach him in as nonthreatening a manner as possible, assuring him privacy and personal space, and keeping demands for verbal responses to a minimum. The nurse can gather valuable data by observation of the client, but the actual process of interviewing may have to be deferred until the client is more comfortable. The establishment of the nurse-client relationship will require spending specific periods of time with the client to indicate the nurse's unqualified interest. Only when the client begins to develop a sense of trust in the nurse can the next step of problem identification occur.

The phenothiazine drugs are among the most frequently used in the treatment of schizophrenic disorders; thus, the nurse should be familiar with the indications, routes of administration, side effects, and nursing measures of these drugs. The hypotension caused by Thorazine is more severe when the drug is administered intramuscularly, and thus it is particularly important to monitor the client's blood pressure and take appropriate precautions. Pseudoparkinsonism is one of the extrapyramidal side effects that occur with the phenothiazine drugs. If this symptom is severe, an antiparkinsonian drug may be prescribed.

QUESTIONS 23-25

The client in crisis has experienced a series of challenges and losses related to her divorce and to the responsibility of dealing with the problems of her children. Most recently she was faced with the additional loss of financial support from her ex-husband.

Review the characteristics of maturational and situational crises and the factors that determine whether an individual will experience a crisis as a result of a stressful event. Review the steps of crisis intervention and the nursing interventions appropriate to each step.

Since crisis intervention is directed toward assisting the client to regain a level of functioning as high as or better than the precrisis level, the nurse should convey an attitude of confidence in the client's ability to work through the present difficulties. When the client has described the precipitating event and how she thinks the problem is affecting her, the nurse can then question the client about how she has coped with problems in the past.

While the nurse may identify resources that the client can call upon for help in her situation, the client is encouraged to make the necessary contacts herself. This further supports the expectation that the client is competent to deal with her problems.

QUESTIONS 26-31

The client's extreme suspiciousness and delusions give evidence of impaired reality testing. This behavior, in combination with intense hostility and assaultiveness, suggests a psychotic disorder of a paranoid type. Since the symptoms of paranoid schizophrenia and paranoid disorders are so similar, it would be useful to review the psychodynamics and prominent defenses of both syndromes.

The self-image of the person who is paranoid is characterized by worthlessness and inadequacy. Early in his life he develops a pattern of disparaging others in an attempt to maintain some self-esteem. He has difficulty in acknowledging the worth of others as well as of himself. He often blames others for his own failures. Because he anticipates rejection from other people, he defends himself by maintaining an emotional distance. Thus, the establishment of a therapeutic relationship with a client such as Mr. Bond requires that the nurse understand his need to avoid interpersonal closeness until he has developed a sense of trust.

When planning care for any client, the nurse must give priority to those areas of functioning that are essential to the integrity and functioning of the individual. In this situation, the problems in maintaining self-control must be addressed first.

Delusions should be neither agreed with nor contradicted by the nurse. Instead, the nurse may use the delusional statement to encourage the client to focus on what is disturbing him.

The disturbance in thinking, known as ideas of reference, is a common symptom in paranoid disorders. The person interprets an event occurring in the environment as having particular significance or reference to himself.

When communicating with a suspicious client, the nurse must be scrupulously honest, consistent, and precise. The nurse should use words that are clear and unambiguous. In an attempt to establish effective communication, the nurse should attempt to clarify the client's statements when they are not clear. This conveys the nurse's interest in understanding the client but does not necessarily indicate agreement. No attempt should be made to disprove the client's delusions by indicating his faulty logic.

The paranoid client's anger and hostility may generate considerable anxiety and negative feelings in the nurse who is working with him. It is important to acknowledge these feelings and to discuss them with other staff members so that they do not become the source of punitive or retaliatory attitudes by the nurse.

## QUESTIONS 32-36

The client's somatic symptoms in the absence of a physical basis are consistent with the diagnosis of somatoform disorder, which used to be classified as a psychoneurotic disorder in the American Psychiatric Association's nomenclature. An essential understanding that the nurse should have in working with the client described is that her symptoms are real and not imaginary. Because the symptoms serve the purpose of reducing the individual's intolerable anxiety and because they are operating on an unconscious level, the client will give up the symptoms only when she has learned a more effective way to deal with the stress she is experiencing.

Review the dynamics of anxiety disorders, somatoform disorders, and dissociative disorders (psychoneurotic disorders, in the older classification system).

Although the nurse may feel frustrated because the client's physical complaints persist in spite of the absence of physio-

logical abnormality, it is most important to convey acceptance of the client as a person as the basis of the therapeutic relationship.

Since anxiety and the methods of coping with anxiety are central to the client's condition, an accurate assessment of her current level of anxiety is necessary in order to plan nursing care. This assessment takes priority over other useful data that the nurse will gather.

Assessing the client's level of anxiety and other feelings she is experiencing is an ongoing process that allows the nurse to take therapeutic action. The client's feelings rather than the nurse's expectations should determine the appropriate intervention.

In question #34 the client evidences phobic behavior by expressing an unfounded fear of elevators. A reflective response to the client's expression of her fears allows the nurse to validate an understanding of the client's communication and also conveys an acceptance of the client's feelings. It is pointless to ask the client why she has this fear, since the origins of the phobia are unconscious and not accessible at this time.

As the client continues to cling to the physiological basis of her somatic complaints, she may challenge the competence of the medical staff or the accuracy of diagnostic tests. The nurse should understand that this behavior is evidence of the difficulty the client has in giving up her defenses against anxiety. The therapeutic response involves a continued acceptance of the client's position rather than an attempt to convince her to abandon it.

In the initial stage of psychotherapy, as clients begin to confront the conflicts that are the source of their symptoms, it is common for them to experience an intensification of anxiety and defensive behavior. The nurse should anticipate this phenomenon.

## QUESTIONS 37-39

Infantile autism, the condition that the 22-month-old child may have, is characterized by severe neurological, perceptual, and behavioral symptoms appearing as early as the first few months of life and before the age of 30 months.

To assess the child, the nurse should have a knowledge of normal childhood growth and development against which to compare the findings obtained.

The child with autistic behavior reveals a disturbance in the development of social relationships. There is often an absence of responsive behavior toward the approach of the parents, and typically the child seems as content alone as in the presence of the parents.

Further indication of the disturbance in the child's capacity for social relationships is his failure to respond to the sound of his parents' voices. As evidence that this occurrence is not caused by a hearing impairment, the child is often particularly attracted to music. The child often demonstrates peculiar motor behavior in the form of spinning, rocking, head-banging, and repetitive arm movements.

Because of the autistic child's avoidance of interpersonal contact and the disturbance in language development that typically occurs, a therapeutic approach to the child offers the nurse's presence without making demands for a response or imposing personal closeness.

## QUESTIONS 40-48

The circumstances of the admission of the client to the alcohol detoxification unit typify the pressures that must be brought to bear upon the client to bring her into treatment. Most commonly it is a family member or employer who issues the ultimatum after the client has had a long period of disturbed functioning related to alcohol consumption.

Review the psychological and social factors that contribute to the development of alcohol abuse. It is important also to consider the theories that propose a contributing biological etiology of alcoholism.

Physiological dependence on alcohol is responsible for the syndrome that occurs when alcohol is withdrawn. The syndrome includes the symptoms of tachycardia, elevated blood pressure, nausea, restlessness, tremors, hallucinations, and convulsions and ultimately may progress to delirium tremens. The client who is being detoxified must be monitored carefully for the development of these symptoms so that adequate measures can be taken to prevent injury, to meet metabolic and nutritional needs, and to minimize anxiety. Although the client in withdrawal may become confused and agitated, the use of physical restraints should be avoided if possible because they tend to increase agitation.

Visual and tactile hallucinations are indicative of the development of delirium tremens. The presence of a staff member offering reassurance and orientation may reduce the client's growing sense of panic and prevent self-injury. The physician should be informed of the client's condition so that the use of a sedative or tranquilizer can be considered.

When a client is in a state of delirium tremens, the potential for physical injury may be so extreme as to be life-threatening, and thus protective measures demand priority.

When the goal of restoration of the client's physiological equilibrium has been met, the psychological problems can be addressed.

It is expected that any client beginning group therapy will experience a period of uncertainty, during which considerable anxiety will be felt. Only when the client has progressed through this phase, and through the phases of overaggression and regression, will she arrive at the adaptation phase, during which she may develop insight into her behavior. It is important to understand the phases through which participants move in group therapy.

One of the treatments that may help an individual maintain abstinence from alcohol is the use of an aversive agent such as disulfiram (Antabuse). The client who takes Antabuse regularly will experience symptoms of nausea, vomiting, and palpitations when even a small amount of alcohol is consumed. The drug is usually used for only a limited time in conjunction with other treatment methods.

Since Alcoholics Anonymous has the most successful record in the treatment of alcoholism, the nurse should be familiar with the methods and philosophy of the organization. Self-help and peer support are offered in an ongoing educational program that assists the member to maintain complete abstinence from alcohol.

The client who is recovering from alcoholism must accept the fact that rehabilitation will require long-term involvement much beyond the phase of "drying-out" or detoxification.

QUESTIONS 49-50

The term "antisocial personality disorder," in the American Psychiatric Association's classification system, has taken the place of the older terms "psychopath" and "sociopath." Review the characteristic behavior and the dynamics that underlie the antisocial personality disorder.

The client's history is typical insofar as it includes drug abuse as well as other illegal and irresponsible activity. Characteristically, the antisocial personality sees other people as objects to be manipulated. He has little concern for the feelings and rights of others and operates on the basis of obtaining immediate gratification of his desires regardless of the consequences. He is often described as lacking an adequate superego or conscience. He seems to feel little remorse for his destructive actions, and he seems unable to learn from experience so as to control his behavior.

In question #50, the client attempts to manipulate the staff by playing one staff member against another. To work effectively with such a client, it is essential for the staff to meet as a group to define treatment goals and to establish a plan of care which must be used consistently by all staff members.

Nurses working with clients with antisocial personality disorders must be aware of the feelings that these clients evoke. Inexperienced nurses especially may be taken in by the superficial charm, apparently clear thinking, and temporary attitude of cooperation shown by the client. When the client's antisocial behavior is again revealed, the nurse may become disappointed and angry and thus unable to function therapeutically with the client until these feelings have been resolved.

The client demonstrates the disturbance in affect, disregard for self-maintenance, and repeated expressions of self-depreciation that are characteristic of a depressed person.

Since the client is not making an independent effort to eat at this time, the nurse must take an active approach in maintaining the client's nutrition. A firm, matter-of-fact manner should be used to inform her of the behaviors that are expected of her, which would include eating a minimum amount of food. The nurse should avoid suggesting that food will provide her with pleasure or will alter the way she feels, as this would negate the client's current perceptions.

The client may express feelings of worthlessness and self-blame, and a need for punishment, which are typical of a severe depression. Rather than trying to argue the client out of her self-view, the nurse should acknowledge her statements without agreeing with them. At this time, the client cannot make a realistic self-appraisal that could help her to set vocational goals. Her extremely low self-esteem can be altered as she experiences small successes in gradually managing the tasks of daily living. The nursing care plan should provide for goals that she can successfully achieve at her current level of functioning.

The nurse should have an understanding of the action of amitriptyline hydrochloride, (Elavil) one of the tricyclic antidepressants used in the treatment of depression. These drugs achieve a therapeutic effect after 14 to 21 days of administration. An accurate evaluation of the client's response to the drug cannot be made until 10 days after beginning the drug.

While the client is encouraged to assume as much responsibility as possible for her self-care, the nurse must be alert for the client's need for assistance in performing tasks. This may be apparent in relation to grooming, particularly in social situations where it would reflect negatively on the client to appear unkempt. Rather than focusing on the client's failure to complete her self-care, the nurse should simply offer assistance.

QUESTIONS 55-58

This situation is another example of a client demonstrating the symptoms of a somatoform disorder.

Question #55 emphasizes the concept that the physical complaints described by the client are as real as those that have a physiologic origin. The primary gain achieved from the symptoms -- the reduction of anxiety -- occurs at an unconscious level. So too does the secondary gain, which may take the form of release from responsibilities because of physical incapacity. It is important to recognize the difference between the nature of the somatic complaints of the somatoform disorder and those of the malingerer who consciously and deliberately feigns illness for some personal gain.

One of the objectives of care for a client with a somatoform disorder is to assist her in identifying and expressing her feelings and needs in a more constructive manner than she is presently doing. This requires planning for adequate time to listen and support her expressions of concern. Because the client appears rational and cooperative, the nurse mistakenly may attempt to use an intellectual, persuasive approach to convince her to abandon her symptoms. Since this approach ignores the dynamics of the condition, it will be of no value.

In order to work effectively with the client, the nurse must shift the focus of attention from the client's physical symptoms to other efforts to cope with her current experience.

## QUESTIONS 59-63

The client's behavior is indicative of an organic mental disorder, a diagnostic term that has replaced the term organic brain syndrome.

Organic mental disorder is a result of the impairment of brain-tissue function caused by any of a wide range of organic factors. Review the etiological categories that have been identified, the differences between acute and chronic disorders, and the characteristic disturbances in behavior.

Diminished sensory perception, common in conditions such as this client's, results in decreased perception of all sensory stimuli. Since she is likely to have a lessened perception of both heat and cold, she will need assistance in dressing appropriately for the environment. Further caution is also necessary to prevent injury from hot water used in bathing, or from other situations involving hot liquids or objects.

One of the goals for the client is to maintain maximum independent functioning in activities of daily living. The client should be encouraged to do as much as possible for herself, but because of her impairment in intellectual functioning, she may require repeated, step-by-step directions to complete such activities as dressing herself. Because of the client's deficits in memory and attention, the nurse should direct the client to the completion of only one component of a task at a time.

The client's ability to cope is affected to a great extent by the demands made by the environment and the support provided within it. While some provision must be made for diversion and stimulation, the daily schedule should be well structured to allow the client to become familiar with the repeated pattern of activities and to minimize the demands for social adaptation.

Clients may be slow in carrying out routine activities because of impairments in orientation and memory and also because of physical disabilities associated with advanced age. Ample time should be allowed for the client to proceed as independently as possible even though this may take more time than if the nurse completed the task for the client.

Hoarding is evidence of the disturbed social behavior that is common to organic mental disorders. The behavior may represent an attempt by the client to deal with irrational fears of being left without food. However,

because the client's intellectual impairment prevents her from comprehending reasonable explanations as to why the hoarding should be discontinued, this approach is of no value. Attempting to remove the hoarded food will create unnecessary stress for the client and may precipitate further dysfunctional behaviors as a response to her frustration. Thus, the most supportive approach is to allow her to keep the food in a hygienic manner.

## QUESTIONS 64-65

While the client is experiencing an attack of acute anxiety, his cognitive functioning is affected so that he is able to attend to only one specific detail at a time. His limited attentiveness interferes with his ability to complete a task or to engage in problem-solving. He needs assistance in reducing his anxiety to a more tolerable level. The nurse can be effective by remaining with the client, maintaining a calm manner, allowing the client to ventilate his feelings, and conveying to him the sense that the nurse will not abandon him. A quiet, restful environment with a minimal number of people can also contribute to the reduction of his anxiety.

Review the definition of anxiety, the levels of anxiety and the behaviors associated with each level, and the functional and dysfunctional mechanisms used in coping with anxiety.

The first step in learning how to cope effectively with anxiety is recognizing that one is anxious. This can be done only when the client has reduced the severe anxiety of an acute episode to a level that allows learning.

QUESTIONS 66-70

The client's mutism, immobility, and sudden bursts of impulsive, purposeless activity are indicative of a schizophrenic disorder. The length of her hospitalization tells us that she is suffering from a chronic form of the disorder. The review of material about schizophrenic disorders that was recommended for questions #19-22 will serve as preparation for the following questions.

The disturbances in language that may occur in schizophrenic disorders include echolalia, clang association, word salad, and neologisms, as well as mutism. Each of these symptoms reflects the disturbances of thinking and the severe regression that are characteristic of the disorder. Language becomes a means the client uses to isolate herself from others so as to protect herself from the anxiety associated with interpersonal closeness.

Clients such as Miss Durby are in such poor contact with reality that they may be totally unaware of their needs for nutrition, rest, and safety. They may seem incapable of carrying out the necessary actions for self-preservation. Thus it becomes essential for the nurse to oversee the client's physical condition and to take appropriate action before other therapeutic interventions can be planned.

Establishing a relationship with a client who has withdrawn into her own private world requires a consistent, patient approach by a nurse who can convey concern and unqualified acceptance. When spending time with Miss Durby, who has been mute, the nurse should attend to and acknowledge the client's nonverbal communication. If the client does express something verbally that is not understandable, it is most important that the nurse convey the desire to understand what the client said. This indicates the nurse's willingness to continue the effort to establish communication with the client, in spite of the difficulties that both persons are experiencing. Encouraging the client to restate her message in a more coherent form is more likely to be therapeutic than a comment that is essentially chit-chat by the nurse.

In question #69 the client is demonstrating the problem of identity confusion. The client has difficulty in conceiving of herself as a total person and also in distinguishing herself from the environment. Because of the client's poor ego boundaries, she may become acutely anxious if someone comes close to her or touches her without warning. The nurse should, therefore, inform the client of the nurse's approach and intentions, and provide information that helps to orient the client to the physical environment. With this client, touch should be used only selectively and with adequate preparation, because the client may interpret touch as a threatening invasion of herself.

When attempting to develop the client's sense of trust, the nurse must be consistent and honest in the relationship with the client, and must fulfill the promises made to the client as much as possible. Being available to the client for scheduled appointments is an indication of the nurse's trustworthiness. There are situations, however, when the nurse's unanticipated absence is unavoidable. The client reacts to such an absence with disappointment and an expression of fear that she will be abandoned by the nurse upon whom she has begun to rely. Rather than trying to minimize the client's reaction or explain the reason for the nurse's absence, the nurse should accept the client's negative feelings and reflect what the nurse believes is inherent in the client's statement. This encourages the client to elaborate further on the feelings that she is experiencing.

## QUESTIONS 71-74

This client, who has an antisocial personality disorder, presents a history that typically includes a number of delinquent acts which the client defends as occurring for some acceptable reason. Typical too is the charming manner and the failure to see his behavior as dysfunctional.

Antisocial behavior such as Mr. Randolph uses to control anxiety is often expressed as an attempt to gain control of others by deception and exploitation, without regard for its destructive consequences. The most therapeutic response to this behavior is the establishment of consistent, reasonable limits by the nurse. These limits should restrict only those actions that are potentially detrimental to the client or to others, and should be presented clearly to the client.

It is common for the client with an antisocial personality disorder to single out a staff member whom he will attempt to manipulate for gratification of his wishes. The nurse must be aware of the client's motivations and of the responses that he may be attempting to elicit from the nurse. The nurse may mistakenly interpet the client's desire to communicate as an expression of real interpersonal closeness; or the nurse may engage in rescue fantasies about saving the client from his destructive behavior. The realistic assessment of the situation is based on the understanding that the nurse can be therapeutically effective only within the established guidelines of the plan of care.

Since one of the deficits that is characteristic of clients with an antisocial personality disorder is the inability to empathize with or feel real concern about another person, the expression of concern shown by the client is a sign of improvement.

Question #74 reinforces the importance of all staff members' working consistently according to an established plan of care and sharing all information about the client. Only when this approach is taken can the client's attempts at manipulation be thwarted.

## QUESTIONS 75-78

The client's history, particularly her impaired judgment and labile affect, suggest that she is suffering from an organic mental disorder. Refer to the material suggested for review for questions 59-63.

Since in many cases the symptoms of organic mental disorder are attributable to systemic illness, nutritional disorders, and the effects of drugs, it is imperative that the client be given a thorough physical examination so that physiologic problems can be addressed.

An improvement in the client's mental status often occurs when the physical problems are treated. With a client such as Mrs. Winter, who has been living as a vagrant, priority must be given to assessing and treating her physical condition, which is probably showing the effects of her recent life-style.

The client demonstrates suspiciousness through her accusations that other people are stealing from her. Any attempt by a staff member to clear away what seems to be useless clutter from the client's belongings is likely to be perceived by her as stealing. Since Mrs. Winter's social judgment and intellectual functioning are impaired, she is unable to respond to requests that she alter her behavior for the sake of greater acceptance by others. The nurse should understand that the client's possessions represent an extension of herself and an affirmation of her personal identity in an alien environment with which she cannot deal effectively. It is most therapeutic to allow the client to use the coping behavior that she has been demonstrating, as long as she is not endangering herself or others.

The client's ability to adapt to a changing

173

environment is markedly impaired because of her intellectual deficits. Thus, to reduce her anxiety in anticipation of a transfer to another facility, a visit to the other facility should be arranged. This would provide her with information that she can absorb more readily than a verbal presentation of what she can expect.

## QUESTIONS 79-82

The client's extreme withdrawal and immobility indicate a psychotic disorder, the precise nature of which has not yet been established, although it is suggestive of a schizophrenic disorder.

The initial assessment of a client such as Mrs. Long, who gives evidence of disturbed verbal communication and impaired contact with reality, must give priority to determining whether she has impulses that would be destructive to herself or others. This assessment will require a period of observation of Mrs. Long's nonverbal behavior, and the gradual encouragement of verbal expression of her thoughts and feelings. Question #79, which illustrates this material, is another example of giving priority to the identification of problems that may be life-threatening.

The client's withdrawal indicates that she is fearful of relatedness with others. She may anticipate being controlled or abandoned by others if she allows herself to break out of her protective shell. Repeated demonstrations of the nurse's interest and reliability, such as providing periods of the nurse's undivided attention, are the basis of the establishment of trust.

The immobility displayed by the client occurs as a result of the extreme anxiety she experiences in anticipation of taking any action. Since she fears the consequences of any action that she may decide to take, she resorts to the defense of no action at all. This behavior does not occur because of insufficient stimulation from the environment. However, the client will usually accept passive exercises since she herself has not chosen to undertake them. As indicated in question #81, these exercises are essential to prevent circulatory and musculoskeletal injury.

The client's diminishing need to maintain interpersonal distance may initially be shown by her ability to tolerate the physical presence of others while not yet engaging in real communication. But the client's willingness to allow greater interpersonal closeness, as she begins to experience trust in the context of the therapeutic relationship, is indicated by eye contact with the nurse.

INDIVIDUAL QUESTIONS 83-98

83. The client who has not been able to regain self-control in response to the staff's initial interventions, and whose agitation has escalated to a level of physical destruction must be considered an immediate threat to himself and others. It is not safe to leave the patient alone for more than a moment or two; nor is it safe to undertake any attempt to control him unless a sufficient number of staff members are present.

84. A self-government group, which is a feature of the therapeutic community, encourages clients to participate in the decision-making that affects the day-to-day operation of the unit. The group promotes the assumption of responsibility as a community member and permits the client's exercise of leadership within a structured setting. However, the nurse who is working with the group must maintain the authority that distinguishes the role of the staff members and must indicate clearly to the clients the limits of the self-government group's responsibility.

85. The client has made a general statement about her fear of dying and her desire to speak to her family. The client's need to express her feelings would be denied by the nurse's offering to speak for the client to her family. This response is presumptuous in that it suggests that the client is incapable of speaking for herself. Furthermore, the nurse has yet to learn what the client is feeling. It is equally nontherapeutic to curtail the client's communication by denying the individuality of her experience, as conveyed by option C. The nurse's insecurity in relating to the client may be expressed by closing off the communication at this time with the suggestion that another staff member will be made available.

A therapeutic response to the client offers an open-ended statement that encourages her to express her thoughts and feelings about the subject she introduced.

86. In this situation the client is expressing a normal grief reaction in response to a significant loss. The nurse should respect her request for privacy at this time and

allow her to grieve, protected from the view of others.

87. The selection of life-saving measures to counteract the effects of drug overdose is dependent on knowing which drug or combination of drugs was used. Other information about the circumstances of the overdose can be useful, but is not as essential.

88. A remotivation program is aimed at increasing the client's awareness of an involvement in the physical and social environment. The use of all senses is encouraged as a means of linking the person to the world around him. Activities should be selected with consideration of the fact that many elderly clients have impairments in sensory perception, and with the goal of enhancing their remaining capacities.

89. One of the primary goals of a client government is the development of a sense of responsibility. This is a level of behavior that goes beyond the skills of planning activities or identifying grievances.

90. A therapeutic response to a client who is experiencing auditory hallucinations requires that the nurse state that the voices are not heard by the nurse. The nurse should not attempt to challenge or argue with the client, but at the same time statements should not be made that suggest that the nurse shares the client's perception.

91. The repeated references to family wealth and prominence, whether real or fabricated, are evidence of the client's attempt to gain self-esteem. Her behavior indicates that in a situation where her self-esteem is diminished, she is resorting to this means of enhancing her image. Recognizing this, the nurse should promote the client's increased self-esteem through other activities that are reality- oriented.

92. The child who is mentally retarded is less able to organize his activities than the average child. He requires that his days be more thoroughly structured by an adult. A familiar routine poses fewer intellectual challenges for the child and allows him greater opportunity to achieve success in his day-to-day activities.

93. The victim of rape is undergoing a crisis; thus, the general goals of crisis intervention are applicable. The client is helped to achieve a pre-crisis level of functioning, which requires restoration of

emotional control so that she is able to deal constructively with the many disturbing feelings that the rape has engendered. Other subsidiary goals may be identified according to the client's individual needs.

94. Anxiety is a feeling that is a necessary and motivating factor when it is experienced in amounts small enough to be used constructively by the individual. The client who has been experiencing severe anxiety must go through a series of steps beginning with the identification of the feeling of anxiety and progressing ultimately to the use of anxiety in a growth-promoting manner.

95. The client's nonverbal behavior conveys his anxiety and difficulty in confronting his altered body image. At this time the nurse can be most therapeutic by accepting and acknowedging his feelings. Rather than focusing on the client's stoma, the nurse indicates regard for him as a person and his individual pace of resolving his loss.

96. The person who is hospitalized, regardless of the diagnosis, is experiencing multiple stresses related to a change in self-concept, isolation from family, loss of independence, physical discomfort, and fear of the implications of one's illness. The person will deal with the stress and anxiety generated by illness in the characteristic way that he or she has used in past stressful situations. It is the individual's personality rather than the seriousness of the illness that most directly determines the coping behavior that is used.

97. An alteration in body structure, such as that which occurs with a hysterectomy, threatens a woman's self-concept. Her adaptation to the loss will depend primarily on her ability to develop a positive reevaluation of her self and her body image. The significance that the woman attaches to the body part, and the meaning that the alteration has in terms of her identity and role, will affect her response to the surgery. Social and cultural factors are secondarily important insofar as they contribute to the woman's self-image.

98. Defense mechanisms may be used by anyone as a means of defending against anxiety. They operate on an unconscious level and are essential for keeping disturbing material out of conscious awareness.

# References for Psychiatric Nursing

Gilman, Alfred Goodman, et al. The
Pharmacological Basis of Therapeutics, 6th
ed. New York: Macmillan Publishing Co.,
1980.

Haber, Judith, et al. Comprehensive
Psychiatric Nursing, 2nd ed. New York:
McGraw-Hill Book Co., 1982.

Rodman, Morton J., and Dorothy W. Smith.
Pharmacology and Drug Therapy in Nursing,
2nd ed. Philadelphia: J. B. Lippincott
Co., 1979.

Stuart, Gail Wiscarz, and Sandra J. Sundeen.
Principles and Practice of Psychiatric
Nursing, 2nd ed. St. Louis, MO: The C. V.
Mosby Co., 1983.

# COMPREHENSIVE TEST
## PART I

Read each question carefully. Select one answer from the four choices presented that you think answers the question correctly. There is only one correct answer to each question. Use the answer key on page 204 to find out whether the answer you selected is the correct one.

Mr. Adam Brown, 67 years old, is seen in the clinic. It is determined that he has early signs of congestive heart failure. A low-sodium diet and a thiazide diuretic are prescribed for him.

1. Since Mr. Brown has congestive heart failure, the nurse should expect that he will most certainly have which of these symptoms?

   A. Distended neck veins.

   B. Shortness of breath.

   C. Stabbing pain in his chest.

   D. Weakness of his leg muscles.

2. To minimize possible side effects of the thiazide diuretic, Mr. Brown should be given which of these instructions?

   A. "Drink at least eight glasses of water every day."

   B. "Take your medication every morning after breakfast."

   C. "Be sure to empty your bladder every two hours."

   D. "Include fresh leafy vegetables or dried fruit in your daily diet."

Two months later, digitalis (Lanoxin) is prescribed for Mr. Brown.

3. Mr. Brown should be taught the symptoms of digitalis toxicity, which include

   A. anorexia.

   B. frontal headache.

   C. bleeding gums.

   D. facial flushing.

4. The primary therapeutic effect of digitalis for Mr. Brown is expected to cause which of these physiological changes?

   A. Improved skin tone.

   B. Increased urinary output.

   C. Strengthened heart contractions.

   D. Decreased respiratory rate.

Mrs. Betty Landon, 46 years old, is admitted to the hospital because of recurring symptoms of cholecystitis.

5. In describing the pain associated with her cholecystitis, Mrs. Landon will most probably say that it radiates to which of these parts of her body?

   A. Left arm.

   B. Right shoulder.

   C. Sacroiliac area of the back.

   D. Left lower quadrant of the abdomen.

6. Mrs. Landon is scheduled for a gallbladder series. In preparation for the test, which of these measures should be carried out for Mrs. Landon the evening before the test?

   A. Administering saline enemas to her until the return is clear.

   B. Serving her a high-fat meal.

   C. Giving her tablets containing a contrast medium.

   D. Having an intravenous infusion started for her.

Test results indicate that Mrs. Landon has cholelithiasis. She has a cholecystectomy, and after a brief stay in the recovery room, she is transferred to her room. She has a nasogastric tube that is attached to low, intermittent suction, and a T-tube that is attached to a drainage bag.

---

Mrs. Barbara Devon, 54 years old, is brought to the psychiatric hospital by her husband. Mrs. Devon has become increasingly depressed and agitated over the past two weeks. Mr. Devon reports that his wife has been eating very little and that she spent the last night pacing and crying.

---

7. Mrs. Landon complains of nausea. Which of these actions should the nurse take first?

   A. Examine Mrs. Landon's abdomen for distention.

   B. Assess the patency of Mrs. Landon's nasogastric tube.

   C. Have Mrs. Landon rinse her mouth with a mild antiseptic solution.

   D. Change Mrs. Landon's position.


8. Mrs. Landon has an intravenous infusion. She is to receive 1,000 ml. of intravenous fluids over an 8-hour period. If 1,000 ml. of fluid is started at 9 a.m., how many milliliters of fluid should have been given by 1 p.m.?

   A. 250

   B. 375

   C. 500

   D. 625


9. On the day of Mrs. Devon's admission to the hospital, priority should be given to which of these measures for her?

   A. Involving her in goal-setting.

   B. Helping her identify her achievements.

   C. Maintaining constant supervision.

   D. Outlining the unit routines.


10. To plan care for Mrs. Devon, which of these assessments will be most important?

   A. How well does Mrs. Devon socialize with other patients?

   B. What thoughts does Mrs. Devon relate?

   C. Does Mrs. Devon have any difficulty making decisions?

   D. Has Mrs. Devon any food preferences?


11. While Mrs. Devon is acutely depressed and agitated, priority should be given to achieving which of these goals?

   A. To have her adhere to daily routines.

   B. To provide psychological support for her.

   C. To maintain her personal hygiene.

   D. To guard her personal safety.

12. In preparation for the electric convulsive therapy, it is important to carry out which of these measures for Mrs. Devon?

    A. Teaching Mrs. Devon how to breathe deeply and cough.

    B. Administering a cleansing enema to Mrs. Devon.

    C. Asking Mrs. Devon if she is allergic to penicillin.

    D. Withholding food and fluids from Mrs. Devon.

13. When the nurse tells Mrs. Devon that it is time to go for the electric convulsive therapy, Mrs. Devon says, "I'm afraid to go." She moves away from the nurse and becomes upset. The nurse should take which of these actions?

    A. Take Mrs. Devon by the hand and walk with her to the treatment area.

    B. Leave Mrs. Devon in her room and report the incident.

    C. Tell Mrs. Devon that her treatment cannot be cancelled at this time.

    D. Remind Mrs. Devon that she signed the consent form.

14. Mrs. Devon has an electric convulsive treatment and she is beginning to respond. Which of these statements should the nurse make first?

    A. "Tell me your name."

    B. "Your treatment is over."

    C. "You will feel better soon."

    D. "Your memory will return gradually."

15. Lisa is to be evaluated for evidence of congenital dysplasia of the hip. The nurse should use which of these methods to assess Lisa for this problem?

    A. Place Lisa on her back, flex her knees, and observe the degree to which each hip can be abducted.

    B. Place Lisa on her abdomen and observe the extension of her hips.

    C. Place Lisa on her abdomen and observe if there is a disparity in the extension of her hips.

    D. Place Lisa on her back, flex her hips, and note if there is a difference between the degree each hip can be adducted.

16. Lisa is to receive her first immunization. In addition to beginning protection against diphtheria, tetanus, and pertussis (DTP), at this time she will most likely receive protection against which of these infectious diseases?

    A. Influenza.

    B. Chicken pox.

    C. Tuberculosis.

    D. Poliomyelitis.

17. In discussing nutrition with the nurse, Mrs. Jacobs says that she typically serves all of the following lunches. Which of these lunches contains foods from each of the basic four food groups?

    A. Hamburger with lettuce and tomato, milk, and banana.

    B. Rice and kidney beans, white bread, apple juice, and ice cream.

    C. Codfish cakes, sweet potato, milk and flavored gelatin.

    D. Tomato soup, wheat crackers, orange juice and applesauce.

18. Mrs. Jacobs says that David started sucking his thumb two months ago. David's thumb sucking is most probably related to

   A. stress.

   B. ambivalence about the baby.

   C. boredom.

   D. a need for attention.

---

When Lisa is 1 year old, the nurse administers the Denver Developmental Screening Test (DDST) to her.

---

19. To obtain the best results on the DDST, the nurse should consider which of these questions?

   A. Does Lisa have a hand preference?

   B. Does Lisa follow directions?

   C. Is Lisa in a good mood?

   D. What is Lisa's weight?

---

Mrs. Wilma Hassen, a 24-year-old salesclerk, visits the antepartal clinic after she has missed three menstrual periods. It is determined that she is about three months pregnant. This is her first pregnancy.

---

20. As part of the initial antepartal physical examination, Mrs. Hassen should have which of these tests?

   A. X-ray pelvimetry.

   B. A urine culture.

   C. A mammography.

   D. Cervical cancer screening.

21. Mrs. Hassen says to the nurse, "Our budget is based on both my husband's and my own salary. Can I continue working in a job that keeps me on my feet all day?" To promote Mrs. Hassen's well-being throughout the pregnancy, the nurse should give Mrs. Hassen which of the following advice?

   A. "You should begin to work part-time."

   B. "You should plan to stop working before your third trimester."

   C. "You will need a sedentary job in the last half of your pregnancy."

   D. "You will probably be able to keep your job throughout your pregnancy."

22. The nurse is reviewing Mrs. Hassen's nutritional needs with her. Which of these combinations of foods will meet Mrs. Hassen's daily requirement for calcium?

   A. One pint of milk and two servings of meat.

   B. One pint of milk, one ounce of cheddar cheese, and one serving of ice cream.

   C. Two eggs and one serving of cottage cheese.

   D. Two servings of leafy green vegetables, one serving of ice cream, and one slice of enriched bread.

23. On Mrs. Hassen's second visit to the antepartal clinic, the results of laboratory tests indicate that she is Rho(D) negative and has an anti-RH titer of 0. Mr. Hassen is Rho(D) positive.

   Based on this information, which of these statements about the Rh status of the fetus is accurate?

   A. Whether the fetus is Rh negative depends on the zygosity of Mr. Hassen.

   B. Whether the fetus is Rh negative depends on the zygosity of Mrs. Hassen.

   C. The fetus has a 25% chance of being Rh negative.

   D. The fetus has a 50% chance of being Rh negative.

Mr. and Mrs. Hassen decide to attend classes that prepare parents for childbirth. They register for a psychoprophylactic (Lamaze) course.

24. The Hassens should be informed that the Lamaze method of preparing women for labor and delivery utilizes which of these techniques?

    A. Behavior modification.

    B. Conditioned reflex.

    C. Scaled reinforcement.

    D. Autosuggestion.

At term, Mrs. Hassen is admitted to the hospital in early active labor. She is accompanied by her husband.

25. Upon admission, Mrs. Hassen has all of the following symptoms. Which one would be <u>LEAST</u> indicative of the onset of true labor?

    A. Blood-tinged mucus from the vagina.

    B. Urinary frequency.

    C. Increase in pelvic pressure.

    D. Regular contractions.

26. Which of these time intervals represents the <u>frequency</u> of Mrs. Hansen's contractions?

    A. From the beginning of one contraction to the end of the next contraction.

    B. From the beginning of one contraction to the beginning of the next contraction.

    C. From the end of one contraction to the beginning of the next contraction.

    D. From the beginning of one contraction to the end of that contraction.

Mrs. Hassen's labor progresses normally, and she delivers spontaneously an apparently normal girl. Mrs. Hassen is transferred to the postpartum unit and Baby Girl Hassen is transferred to the newborn nursery.

27. During the "taking-in" phase of the puerperium, Mrs. Hassen should be expected to display which of these behaviors?

    A. Poor appetite, concern over her excretory functions, and irritability.

    B. Shyness, disinterest in surroundings, and ambivalence toward the baby.

    C. Taking responsibility for her own self-care, eagerness to care for the baby, and unwillingness to listen to advice from others.

    D. Resting, compliance with requests from others, and need to talk about her labor experience.

Judy Lasser, 5 years old, is admitted to the hospital with an exacerbation of symptoms of acute lymphocytic leukemia, which was diagnosed a year ago.

28. Judy has had frequent venipunctures during the past year. In preparation for a venipuncture at this time, the nurse should have which of these expectations of Judy's behavior?

    A. Judy's acceptance of the procedure is in direct proportion to the thoroughness of the explanation that Judy receives each time.

    B. Judy's acceptance of the procedure depends on the experience of the nurse who assists with such a procedure.

    C. Judy's acceptance of the procedure is affected more by the length of time that she has had the disease than by her age.

    D. Judy's previous experience with the procedure does not necessarily mean that she will accept it the next time it is done.

---
Judy receives a cytotoxic drug.
---

29. While Judy receives cytotoxic drug therapy,
    she will probably develop which of these
    side effects?

    A. Tinnitus.

    B. Hirsutism.

    C. Alopecia.

    D. Syncope.

30. Judy develops ulcerations on the oral
    mucosa. Which of these breakfasts would be
    most suitable for her?

    A. Orange juice, shredded wheat, and milk.

    B. Apple juice, oatmeal, and chocolate milk.

    C. Cornflakes, fresh strawberries, and
       cocoa.

    D. Bacon strips, buttered toast, and milk.

---
Judy's condition improves, and she is being
prepared for discharge.
---

31. Before this hospitalization, Judy attended
    nursery school. Judy's mother says to the
    nurse, "Well, I guess this ends Judy's
    nursery school... and she loves it so
    much." The nurse should give Judy's mother
    which of the following information about
    appropriate activity for Judy at this time?

    A. Judy's usual activities, including
       nursery school, should be continued as
       long as she is able to manage them.

    B. Judy's physical activity will need to be
       limited, and she will require extra rest
       periods.

    C. Judy's mother should ask the nursery
       school teacher about activities that can
       be continued at home.

    D. Judy's intellectual development will be
       slowed by her illness, and this
       limitation must be considered.

---
When Judy is 6 1/2 years old, she is readmitted
to the hospital with an exacerbation of the
symptoms of acute lymphocytic leukemia. She is
in critical condition, and she dies a few days
after admission.
---

32. Judy's father asks the nurse how he should
    explain her death to their 5-year-old. The
    nurse should tell him that 5-year-olds
    typically conceive of death as

    A. prolonged sleep.

    B. flight from unknown enemies.

    C. transformation from one type of life to
       another.

    D. nothingness.

---
Mrs. Anna Davis, 80 years old, is admitted to
the hospital following a cerebrovascular
accident. She responds verbally to questions,
but she is unable to move her left side. Her
orders include intravenous therapy.
---

33. On admission, Mrs. Davis is placed on her
    right side. This position will achieve
    which of these purposes initially?

    A. To promote her comfort.

    B. To avoid pressure on her affected side.

    C. To increase the depth of her
       respirations.

    D. To maintain patency of her airway until
       her ability to swallow is assessed.

34. Mrs. Davis's intravenous drop rate should
    be monitored carefully to prevent which of
    these complications?

    A. Phlebitis.

    B. Renal overload.

    C. Pulmonary edema.

    D. Hepatic failure.

35. To prevent foot drop in Mrs. Davis's affected extremity, it is most important to carry out which of these exercises?

A. Wiggling her toes.

B. Flexing her knee.

C. Rotating her ankle.

D. Turning her foot from side to side.

36. When care is given to Mrs. Davis, she tells the nurse how to carry out each measure. Which of these interpretations of this behavior would serve as the best basis for planning an approach by the nurse?

A. Mrs. Davis is attempting to maintain her autonomy.

B. Mrs. Davis is demonstrating a return to more child-like actions.

C. Mrs. Davis is exhibiting a lack of confidence in the staff.

D. Mrs. Davis requires an explanation about the procedures being performed.

---

Mrs. Davis's condition becomes stable, but she continues to be paralyzed on her left side. She is out of bed in a chair, and her diet prescription permits foods as tolerated.

---

37. At this time, it would be most important to include which of these measures in Mrs. Davis's daily care?

A. Encouraging her to remain out of bed as long as possible.

B. Providing opportunities for her to socialize.

C. Discussing with her ways in which she can deal with her permanent disability.

D. Teaching her exercises that may restore the function of her affected side.

38. As a result of the normal aging process, Mrs. Davis most probably has which of these physiological alterations?

A. Intestinal hypermotility.

B. Decreased metabolic rate.

C. Disinterest in the opposite sex.

D. Intolerance of foods containing lactose.

---

Mr. Peter Cannon, 60 years old, is admitted to the hospital because it is suspected that he has a tumor of the left lung. He has a bronchoscopy.

---

39. Immediately after the bronchoscopy, which of these measures is important in Mr. Cannon's care?

A. Taking his pulse every half hour.

B. Encouraging him to cough.

C. Giving him ice chips by mouth.

D. Monitoring his respirations.

---

The results of the diagnostic studies confirm that Mr. Cannon has a tumor in the left lung, and a segmental resection of his left lower lobe is performed. During surgery, two chest tubes are inserted and attached to a waterseal drainage system. When his condition is stable, Mr. Cannon is transferred to his room. He is to be out of bed in a chair once a day.

---

40. Mr. Cannon is observed for the earliest symptom of hypoxia, which includes

A. lethargy.

B. cyanosis.

C. restlessness.

D. nystagmus.

41. Mr. Cannon is to be assisted in deep-breathing and coughing every three hours. The primary purpose of this measure for him is to

A. increase the drainage of secretions from his wound.

B. stimulate the respiratory center in the brain.

C. promote re-expansion of his affected lung.

D. liquefy secretions in his respiratory tract.

42. The care of Mr. Cannon's chest drainage system should include which of these measures?

A. Checking that the fluid in the long waterseal tube is fluctuating with his respirations.

B. Irrigating the drainage tubing with sterile saline solution.

C. Clamping the chest tubes when assisting him in coughing.

D. Applying an antibiotic ointment to the insertion sites of the chest tubes.

---------------------------------------------------
Mrs. Sally Mann, 32 years old, is brought to the psychiatric hospital by her husband. This is her second admission. Mr. Mann states that his wife has refused to take her prescribed lithium carbonate for the past month. Two weeks ago she went on a shopping spree and charged expensive gifts that she sent to friends and relatives. Yesterday she told the neighbors that they needed a new car, and she ordered one for them. Mrs. Mann has also spent hours making random telephone calls asking people to join a social club she is planning to organize. Mrs. Mann has lost weight because she has not had time to eat or to sleep. She is admitted to the psychiatric unit.
---------------------------------------------------

43. When the nurse assigned to care for Mrs. Mann approaches her, Mrs. Mann says, "You're new here. I know my way around this place. I'm going to arrange a big party here for everyone to have a good time. Want to help me?" The nurse should make which of these responses to Mrs. Mann?

A. "You sound very cheerful, Mrs. Mann."

B. "Hello, Mrs. Mann, I am your nurse today."

C. "Slow down, Mrs. Mann. You need to talk with the social committee on this unit."

D. "Let's go and talk, Mrs. Mann. I want you to tell me about yourself."

44. Mrs. Mann is hyperactive and expresses many ideas in rapid sequence. To communicate with Mrs. Mann, the nurse should use which of these approaches?

A. Get her attention and be brief.

B. Tell her to be quiet and have her repeat instructions.

C. Wait for a pause in her monologue and comment on her last statement.

D. Tell her that she is wearing herself out and insist that she remain quiet for ten minutes.

45. While Mrs. Mann is acutely ill, priority should be given to which of these goals of care?

A. To prevent her from becoming the center of attention.

B. To meet her physical needs.

C. To prevent her from confronting other patients.

D. To establish a therapeutic relationship with her.

46. Mrs. Mann criticizes the nurse caring for her without having just cause. The nurse should take which of these actions?

A. Request that another staff member be assigned to Mrs. Mann.

B. Overlook Mrs. Mann's comments.

C. Explain to Mrs. Mann why her statements are ojectionable.

D. Tell Mrs. Mann that she is jealous.

47. Mrs. Mann has poor eating habits, and she has a weight loss of about 4 lb. (2 kg.) in one week. Which of these measures is most likely to result in Mrs. Mann's gaining weight?

A. Serving her foods that are in sealed containers.

B. Serving a diet high in calories.

C. Adding snacks between meals and at bedtime.

D. Having her select the foods she prefers.

48. Mrs. Mann's condition improves, and she is to participate in group therapy. A desired outcome of group therapy for her is to

A. gain understanding of her interaction with people.

B. participate in a structured program.

C. learn to listen to others.

D. discover what motivates her behavior.

---------------------------------------------------
Miss Angela Barton, a 15-year-old high school junior, attends a clinic for adolescents who are pregnant. Mrs. Barton, her mother, accompanies Angela to the clinic for the first visit. Angela is 3 months pregnant. This is her first pregnancy.
---------------------------------------------------

49. To help Mrs. Barton understand Angela's actions during her pregnancy, the nurse should explain to Mrs. Barton that Angela will probably behave in which of these ways?

A. She will mature rapidly as a result of the responsibilities of her situation.

B. She will use her mother as a role model.

C. She will ask friends rather than her mother for help in making decisions.

D. She will vacillate between being independent and being dependent.

---------------------------------------------------
Miss Barton attends the clinic regularly. When she is in the 8th month of pregnancy, her blood pressure is elevated and she has proteinuria. She is admitted to the hospital with pregnancy-induced hypertension.
---------------------------------------------------

50. The onset of eclampsia in Miss Barton would be indicated by which of these symptoms?

A. Convulsions.

B. Edema of the hands and feet.

C. Painless vaginal bleeding.

D. Continuous cramps in the lower abdomen.

51. Miss Barton is receiving magnesium sulfate. Because of the possibility of toxic effects from this drug, it is essential to assess her

A. pupillary reaction to light.

B. blood pressure.

C. deep tendon reflexes.

D. specific gravity of urine.

Miss Barton goes into labor, and the labor progresses satisfactorily. She has an episiotomy and delivers a girl. She is transferred to the postpartum unit, and Baby Girl Barton is transferred to the nursery.

52. Because of Miss Barton's symptoms prior to labor, she needs to be observed closely in the early postpartum period for signs of

A. cystitis.

B. thrombophlebitis.

C. nephritis.

D. seizures.

53. Baby Girl Barton is assessed as having a gestational age of 36 weeks. Which of these findings is in keeping with this gestational age?

A. Leathery, wrinkled skin.

B. Deep creases covering the soles of the feet.

C. Ears that lie flat against the skull.

D. Fingernails that are long and brittle.

Baby Girl Barton is to be gavage-fed.

54. To promote gastric emptying after feedings, Baby Girl Barton should be placed in which of these positions?

A. On her right side.

B. On her side with her head lower than her body.

C. On her back, with her head elevated about 45 degrees.

D. On her abdomen, with her head turned to the side.

55. On Miss Barton's first postpartum morning, she is quiet and indecisive. She seems to want the nurse who is taking care of her to do everything for her. Based on this information, which of these interpretations of Miss Barton's behavior is most justifiable?

A. It reflects the taking-in phase of adjustment.

B. It suggests a poor potential for maternal-infant bonding.

C. It indicates an impending postpartum depression.

D. It demonstrates an inability to terminate the symbiotic relationship with the infant.

Miss Barton is discharged on her fourth postpartum day. Baby Girl Barton is discharged when she is two weeks old.

56. When Miss Barton returns to the clinic for a 6-week postpartum checkup, she has an intrauterine device (IUD) inserted. Which of the following information about having an IUD should she be given?

A. She will require a reinsertion in 3 months.

B. She may have menstrual flow that is lighter than usual.

C. She will require a pelvic x-ray in a month.

D. She may have cramping during the next day or two.

---
Mrs. Rena Engle, a 78-year-old widow, falls on the walk in front of her house. A neighbor who is a nurse observes the incident and goes to Mrs. Engle's assistance. The nurse suspects that Mrs. Engle has a fracture of the right femur and calls for an ambulance.

---

57. Early indications of a hip fracture in Mrs. Engle will probably include which of these observations of the affected extremity?

A. Marked swelling.

B. Hematoma.

C. Sudden onset of pallor.

D. Abnormal position.

58. Before the ambulance arrives, it would be essential for the nurse to take which of these actions for Mrs. Engle?

A. Determine if Mrs. Engle has sustained other injuries.

B. Assist Mrs. Engle into a protected area.

C. Leave Mrs. Engle as she is.

D. Give Mrs. Engle sips of warm fluid.

---
Mrs. Engle is taken to the hospital by ambulance. The results of x-rays reveal a fracture of the neck of the right femur. Mrs. Engle is admitted to a surgical unit, and skin traction (Buck's extension) is applied to her affected extremity. She is scheduled to have a surgical repair of the fracture.

---

59. The nurse observes that the weights of Mrs. Engle's traction are close to the floor. The nurse should take which of these actions?

A. Increase the elevation of the head of the bed.

B. Shorten the ropes of the traction.

C. Assist Mrs. Engle to move up in bed.

D. Place a pillow under Mrs. Engle's right heel.

60. The primary purpose of skin traction for Mrs. Engle is to

A. decrease edema in the injured extremity.

B. immobilize the fracture.

C. initiate union of the fracture.

D. promote blood supply to the injured extremity.

---
Mrs. Engle has a pinning of her right hip. When she is transferred to the surgical unit, she has an intravenous infusion. She is to be out of bed in a chair on her first postoperative day.

---

61. Mrs. Engle should be observed for early symptoms of circulatory overload by making which of these assessments?

A. Monitoring her blood pressure.

B. Taking her temperature every 4 hours.

C. Measuring her urinary output.

D. Auscultating her chest.

62. After Mrs. Engle is transferred from the bed to a chair, it would be most important for the nurse to take which of these actions?

A. Compare the pulse in Mrs. Engle's lower extremities.

B. Tell Mrs. Engle to place both feet firmly on the floor.

C. Check Mrs. Engle's heart rate.

D. Secure Mrs. Engle in her seat with a body restraint.

63. To assess Mrs. Engle's bowel function, it would be most important to obtain which of the following information about her usual bowel habits?

A. The laxative she takes to have a bowel movement.

B. The number of bowel movements she has daily.

C. The consistency of each of her bowel movements.

D. The regularity of her bowel movements.

---

Mr. Kenneth Furman, a 40-year-old accountant, is admitted to the hospital with a possible right renal calculus. His orders include an intravenous pyelogram (IVP) and diet as tolerated.

---

64. Mr. Furman's preparation for the IVP should include which of these measures?

A. Collecting a 24-hour urine specimen.

B. Obtaining a history of allergies.

C. Measuring each voiding.

D. Withholding foods containing calcium.

---

The results of the IVP reveal that Mr. Furman has a calculus in the pelvis of the right kidney. He is prepared for a right nephrolithotomy. His preoperative orders include atropine sulfate and meperidine (Demerol) hydrochloride.

---

65. Atropine is administered to Mr. Furman to achieve which of these purposes?

A. To depress the central nervous system.

B. To decrease secretions of the respiratory tract.

C. To stimulate peripheral circulation.

D. To increase the tone of smooth muscles.

---

Mr. Furman has a right nephrolithotomy. After a stay in the recovery room, he is returned to his room.

---

66. Postoperatively, Mr. Furman should be turned frequently for the purpose of preventing

A. respiratory complications.

B. suppression of urine.

C. deformities of the ureters.

D. stasis of urine in the kidney.

67. A diet as tolerated is ordered for Mr. Furman. To promote wound healing, Mr. Furman should be encouraged to eat foods that are high in which of these vitamins?

A. A

B. $B_6$

C. C

D. K

---

Mr. Furman's condition improves, and he is being prepared for discharge.

---

68. To prevent the recurrence of renal calculi, it is most important that Mr. Furman include which of these measures in his daily care?

A. Eating foods high in protein.

B. Emptying his bladder q. 2h.

C. Exercising regularly.

D. Drinking large amounts of fluid.

Susan Anderson, 4 1/2 years old, is attending the pediatric cardiology clinic. Susan has a ventricular septal defect and is to be admitted to the hospital in 2 weeks for surgical repair of her cardiac anomaly.

69. Since Susan has a ventricular septal defect, she has which of these physiological alterations?

A. The blood is shunted from the left to the right ventricle.

B. The left ventricle enlarges to accommodate an increased volume of blood.

C. The pressure is decreased in an abnormally dilated pulmonary artery.

D. The pressure in the right side of the heart is greater than the pressure in the left side.

70. In preparation for Susan's hospitalization, the nurse should give Mrs. Anderson which of these instructions?

A. "Avoid arguments that may upset Susan."

B. "Keep Susan away fron anyone who has a respiratory infection."

C. "Arrange for Susan to play alone for at least two hours each day."

D. "Encourage Susan to drink at least a quart of orange juice each day."

Susan is admitted to the hospital as scheduled.

71. The nurse is preparing Susan for her surgical experience. Because of a fear common to 4-year-old children, it is essential to stress which of these ideas to Susan?

A. She will be able to walk within a few days after surgery.

B. She will not be awake during the operative procedure.

C. Only her heart is to be operated on.

D. She can have medication to relieve pain postoperatively.

72. Susan is to be given preoperative medications intramuscularly. Before giving an intramuscular injection to a child of Susan's age, it is essential to take which of these measures?

A. Having another person available to hold Susan while the injection is given.

B. Showing Susan the syringe and needle to be used for the injection.

C. Asking Susan the site where she would like the injection to be given.

D. Encouraging Susan to remember if she has ever had an injection before.

Susan has a surgical repair of her ventricular
septal defect. On her second postoperative
day, she is transferred to the pediatric unit
from the cardiac intensive care unit. Her
chest tube has been removed. She is receiving
an intravenous infusion through a vein in her
left leg. Mrs. Anderson is with Susan.

73. Soon after Susan is transferred, she starts
to cry and asks her mother to pick her up.
The nurse should take which of these
actions?

A. Help to place Susan on her mother's lap.

B. Ask Mrs. Anderson what she usually does
to comfort Susan.

C. Suggest that Mrs. Anderson leave the
room until Susan calms down.

D. Explain to Mrs. Anderson and Susan that
Susan must stay on bed rest while
receiving intravenous therapy.

Cindy Devon, 4 years old, is admitted to the
hospital with nephrosis.

74. Cindy's initial symptom of nephrosis was
primarily caused by which of these
pathological alterations?

A. Ischemia of the renal cortex.

B. Inflammation of the renal tubules.

C. Decreased level of antidiuretic hormone.

D. Increased permeability of the glomerular
membrane.

75. The morning after Cindy was admitted, she
says to the nurse, "Get out! I don't want
you." The nurse's response should include
which of these statements?

A. "You don't like me."

B. "It's all right for you to be angry."

C. "I want to take care of you."

D. "I'm sorry that you don't like me."

76. Cindy is able to be out of bed for most of
the day. Considering her age and her
condition, which of these play activities
would probably be most suitable for her?

A. Listening to stories.

B. Playing hide-and-go-seek.

C. Using a pounding board.

D. Cutting out paper dolls.

77. Cindy is to receive prednisone by mouth.
The purpose of prednisone for her is to

A. reduce excretion of protein.

B. improve the circulation to her kidney.

C. decrease her blood pressure.

D. stimulate adrenocortical production.

78. Cindy begins to diurese. Since she will
probably have an electrolyte disturbance at
this time, she should be served which of
these snacks?

A. Flavored gelatin.

B. Unsalted pretzels.

C. Orange juice.

D. Buttered popcorn.

79. One morning, Cindy asks the nurse, "When is
my mommy coming?" Mrs. Devon had informed
the nurse that she would be arriving at
about 1:30 p.m. The nurse should give
Cindy which of these answers?

A. "Your mommy will come after you play for
a while and have your lunch."

B. "Your mommy is coming later today."

C. "Let me show you on my watch the time
your mommy will be here."

D. "Your mommy will be here after she gets
her housework done."

Harry Ogdan, 16 years old, arrives in the emergency room and asks to speak to a nurse about a personal problem. The nurse takes Harry to a room that provides privacy.

80. Harry tells the nurse that he suspects he has gonorrhea. The nurse should determine if Harry has a symptom common in males who have gonorrhea, which is

    A. hematuria.

    B. scrotal tenderness.

    C. ulceration on the penis.

    D. purulent urethral discharge.

81. Since Harry is a minor, the nurse should have which of these understandings about the legality of treating a minor who has venereal disease?

    A. Consent for treatment is required from a parent or guardian.

    B. Consent for treatment for venereal disease is not required from a parent or guardian.

    C. Consent for treatment may be given by a minor after signing a release that removes liability from persons giving the treatment.

    D. Consent for treatment from a parent or guardian may be obtained after the treatment is given.

Harry has gonorrhea. His treatment includes penicillin intramuscularly and probenecid (Benemid) orally.

82. Benemid is given to Harry for which of these purposes?

    A. To block renal excretion of penicillin.

    B. To prevent an allergic reaction to penicillin.

    C. To promote rapid metabolism of the penicillin.

    D. To facilitate the transport of penicillin across cell membranes.

83. Before Harry leaves the emergency room, he should be given which of the following information about self-care?

    A. He should increase his intake of fluids for a few days.

    B. He should shower rather than take a tub bath for several days.

    C. He should cleanse his penis with soap and water after each voiding.

    D. He should return to the clinic for an examination in one week.

Mrs. Mabel Young, 38 years old, is brought to the psychiatric hospital by her husband. Mrs. Young was always proud of being a meticulous housekeeper. For the past two months, her cleaning activities are consuming all her time and preventing her from fulfilling other responsibilities. She insists that everyone entering the house remove their shoes, and she places towels on chairs where anyone wants to sit. She scrubs and cleans during the day, and after the family has gone to bed, she begins to clean everything again. Mrs. Young is admitted to the psychiatric unit.

84. Mrs. Young's repeated cleaning activities are most directly related to which of these problems?

A. Her lack of diversional interests.

B. Her need for excellence.

C. Her fear of infections.

D. Her anxiety level.

85. When the nurse enters Mrs. Young's room, Mrs. Young has just finished scrubbing the sink. The nurse talks with Mrs. Young for two minutes, and Mrs. Young starts to scrub the sink again. To meet Mrs. Young's need at this time, the nurse should take which of these actions?

A. Ask Mrs. Young to delay cleaning the sink until they have finished their conversation.

B. Allow Mrs. Young to continue cleaning the sink without making any comment.

C. Remind Mrs. Young that she just finished cleaning the sink.

D. Make a statement to Mrs. Young that suggests a reason for her need to clean the sink.

86. One of the most important plans for Mrs. Young's nursing care in the hospital is

A. preparing her for any changes in her routines.

B. discussing her favorite topic with her while she is carrying out her rituals.

C. preventing her from carrying out her rituals.

D. engaging her in activities that require little or no attention.

87. Mrs. Young is scheduled to participate in activities planned for patients on the unit. She is frequently not prepared to participate because she is carrying out her cleaning rituals. To promote Mrs. Young's participation in activities, the nurse should take which of these actions?

A. Plan individual activities for Mrs. Young to perform when she is ready.

B. Remain with Mrs. Young while she gets dressed before the activity.

C. Give Mrs. Young several reminders of the time for the scheduled activity.

D. Schedule a unit conference so that patients can tell Mrs. Young their reactions to delaying their activities.

Mrs. Jane Cole, 23 years old, is 3 months pregnant. She has had diabetes mellitus for the past 5 years and is taking isophane (NPH) insulin. She is attending an antepartal diabetic clinic. This is Mrs. Cole's first pregnancy.

88. Which of these findings is a normal physiological change of pregnancy that may affect the determination of insulin requirements for Mrs. Cole?

A. An increase in the carbon dioxide content of the plasma.

B. A marked decrease in the secretion of glucagon.

C. A progressive decrease in free fatty acids in the blood.

D. A decreased renal threshold for sugar.

89. Mrs. Cole is instructed to divide her daily food intake so that she can have snacks throughout the day and at bedtime. This pattern of food intake is suggested for which of these purposes?

A. To minimize gastric distention.

B. To maintain stable serum glucose levels.

C. To control weight gain.

D. To regulate the rate of insulin production.

--------------------------------------------------
Mrs. Cole is now in her 6th month of gestation.
--------------------------------------------------

90. Mrs. Cole complains of leg cramps. Which of these exercises may be recommended to relieve leg cramps?

A. Abducting the legs and plantar-flexing the feet.

B. Everting the feet and rotating the legs externally.

C. Dorsiflexing the feet and extending the legs.

D. Inverting the feet and adducting the legs.

91. Mrs. Cole complains of occasional low back pain. The nurse should take which of these measures?

A. Showing her how to apply pressure to the sacral area.

B. Advising her to take frequent short walks.

C. Encouraging her to sit only in straight-backed chairs.

D. Teaching her isometric exercises.

--------------------------------------------------
Mrs. Cole is in the third trimester of pregnancy.
--------------------------------------------------

92. In the third trimester of pregnancy, the nurse should give anticipatory guidance to Mrs. Cole in dealing with which of these developmental tasks?

A. Accepting feelings of ambivalence toward pregnancy.

B. Relinquishing attachment to one's own mother.

C. Conceptualizing the infant as a separate being in need of care.

D. Incorporating the infant into the family structure.

93. Mrs. Cole develops a monilial infection. It is important that the infection be treated to prevent which of these problems in the newborn?

A. Cradle cap.

B. Thrush.

C. Erythema toxicum.

D. Ophthalmia neonatorum.

94. Mrs. Cole has an amniocentesis done at 37 weeks' gestation. The lecithin/ sphingomyelin (L/S) ratio is 2:1; the creatinine value is 2 mg. per 100 ml. Based on these findings, if the baby were born at this time, the baby would definitely have a need for

A. supplemental oxygen therapy.

B. tracheal intubation.

C. gastric decompression.

D. a warm environment.

---
Mrs. Cole's labor is to be induced at 37 weeks' gestation by the use of oxytocin.
---

95. The chief purpose of preterm induction of labor for a woman who has diabetes mellitus is to deliver the fetus before which of these complications occurs?

    A. Hypoglycemia.

    B. Pregnancy-induced hypertension.

    C. Placental insufficiency.

    D. Uterine inertia.

---
Mrs. Cole is given an oxytocin. Her labor is electronically monitored.
---

96. At which of these times should Mrs. Cole's oxytocin infusion be discontinued?

    A. When relaxation between contractions is insufficient for placental perfusion.

    B. When contractions occur every 3 minutes.

    C. When contractions result in a change in fetal station.

    D. When contractions occur in which the increment is longer than the acme.

---
Mrs. Barbara Norman, 20 years old, is seen in the emergency room for treatment of a severe asthmatic attack. She is dyspneic and wheezing.
---

97. The goals of treatment for Mrs. Norman should include reversing which of these pathophysiological alterations?

    A. Atrophy of alveoli.

    B. Pulmonary vasodilatation.

    C. Production of tenacious mucus.

    D. Edema of the larynx.

98. Mrs. Norman is taught to use a nebulizer with isoproterenol (Isuprel) hydrochloride p.r.n. The purpose of this treatment is to

    A. restore the action of the cilia in the bronchi.

    B. suppress the neural receptors in the respiratory center.

    C. increase the tone of respiratory muscles.

    D. relax the smooth muscle of the bronchi.

---
Mrs. Norman's condition improves, and one week later she is seen in the medical clinic.
---

99. The physician prescribes an aminophylline suppository p.r.n. for Mrs. Norman. The purpose of this medication is to

    A. improve the compliance of her lungs.

    B. promote venous circulation in her respiratory tract.

    C. increase her chest expansion.

    D. dilate her bronchi.

100. Mrs. Norman tells the nurse that lately she has been using her isoproterenol (Isuprel) hydrochloride nebulizer every two hours. Excessive use of Isuprel may cause which of these side effects?

    A. Mental depression.

    B. Diarrhea.

    C. Rapid heart rate.

    D. Constriction of peripheral blood vessels.

101. Mrs. Norman says that when she gets up in the morning, she has spasms of coughing and expectorates thick sputum. The nurse should encourage Mrs. Norman to include which of these measures in her daily care?

A. Eating a few crackers before getting out of bed.

B. Moving slowly upon arising.

C. Using a lemon-and-salt solution for oral hygiene.

D. Increasing the humidity in her bedroom with a pan of water.

---

A month later Mrs. Norman reports that her asthma is getting worse. She says that she is having difficulty sleeping and performing her daily activities.

---

102. Prednisone is ordered for Mrs. Norman. The desired effect of this medication for her is to

A. reduce the severity of her symptoms.

B. relieve her anxiety.

C. accelerate the rate of oxygen-carbon dioxide exchange.

D. counteract the side effects of other medications she is taking.

103. While Mrs. Norman is receiving prednisone, she should include which of these measures in her care?

A. Taking her pulse following physical exercise.

B. Using salt liberally on food.

C. Protecting herself from infection.

D. Applying a bland lotion to her skin after bathing.

---

Miss Grace Neuman, 16 years old, takes lessons in driving a car. On the day she is scheduled to take the driving test for her license, she awakens unable to move her right arm and right leg. She is admitted to the hospital. Diagnostic tests reveal no organic basis for Miss Neuman's paralysis. Miss Neuman is transferred to the psychiatric unit.

---

104. When Miss Neuman is admitted to the psychiatric unit, the nurse should initiate a relationship with Miss Neuman by using which of these approaches?

A. Expressing concern to Miss Neuman about the effects of her paralysis.

B. Displaying interest in Miss Neuman without focusing on her disability.

C. Encouraging Miss Neuman to explore her fear of driving a car.

D. Discussing with Miss Neuman her experiences while in a moving vehicle.

105. Since Miss Neuman has hemiplegia of the right·side, her care plan should include which of these measures?

A. Meeting her needs as for any patient who has paralysis.

B. Helping her to accept the loss of body functions.

C. Urging her to move the affected extremities.

D. Encouraging her to consider the lack of evidence of physical trauma.

106. The nurse should expect Miss Neuman to display which of these attitudes about her hemiplegia?

A. She will ignore the disability resulting from the paralysis.

B. She will demonstrate unconcern about the loss of function.

C. She will refuse assistance from the staff members.

D. She will begin to display signs of the grieving process.

107. When Miss Neuman is sitting in a wheelchair in the dayroom, other patients express concern over her disability and are very solicitous of Miss Neuman. Miss Neuman enjoys this attention from them. To provide a therapeutic climate for Miss Neuman, the nurse should consider taking which of these approaches in this situation?

A. Advising the patients that Miss Neuman's disability is the result of emotional conflicts.

B. Helping Miss Neuman to become independent of assistance from other patients.

C. Encouraging non-helping aspects of Miss Neuman's relationship with other patients.

D. Assessing the satisfactions other patients achieve in being helpful to Miss Neuman.

-----------------------------------------------

Mr. Ralph Miller, 61 years old, is admitted to the hospital for a transurethral resection of the prostate. He has a benign hypertrophy of the prostate gland.

-----------------------------------------------

108. Mr. Miller makes all of the following statements. Which one is related to his present condition?

A. "I passed a kidney stone two years ago."

B. "I do not drink milk or eat cheese."

C. "My job requires me to stand most of the day."

D. "My urine has started to look cloudy."

109. The results of Mr. Miller's urinalysis indicate a specific gravity of 1.028. The nurse should most certainly take which of these actions?

A. Encourage Mr. Miller to increase his fluid intake.

B. Offer Mr. Miller cranberry juice between meals.

C. Initiate an intake and output record for Mr. Miller.

D. Check the results of Mr. Miller's blood tests.

110. Mr. Miller is scheduled to have an intravenous pyelogram. His preparation will most probably include which of these measures?

A. Administering tablets containing contrast medium.

B. Collecting fractional urine specimens.

C. Serving fat-free meals before the test.

D. Cleansing the large bowel.

-----------------------------------------------

Mr. Miller has a transurethral resection of the prostate. When he is brought to his room, he has an indwelling urethral catheter attached to gravity drainage.

-----------------------------------------------

111. During the first postoperative night, Mr. Miller becomes restless and begins to pull on his catheter. The nurse should take which of these actions?

A. Obtain an order for a sedative for Mr. Miller.

B. Check the patency of Mr. Miller's urinary drainage system.

C. Inform Mr. Miller that contaminating the catheter will cause an infection.

D. Restrain Mr. Miller's wrists so that he cannot reach the catheter.

Mr. Miller's postoperative progress is good. The urinary catheter is removed, and Mr. Miller is being prepared for discharge.

112. When Mr. Miller's catheter is removed, which of these measures is most important?

    A. Monitoring the time and amount of each voiding.

    B. Encouraging ambulation.

    C. Increasing intake of fluids by mouth.

    D. Determining residual urine after each voiding.

113. Mr. Miller complains of dribbling urine which he cannot control. The nurse's response to Mr. Miller should include which of these statements?

    A. "When you finish urinating, wait a minute and try to urinate again."

    B. "Begin to tighten and relax your buttocks several times a day to strengthen your perineal muscles."

    C. "Your problem is due to a bladder infection that will last for a few days."

    D. "It is an expected occurrence that will continue until the healing is complete."

Mrs. Emily Patterson, 55 years old, is attending the clinic because she has glaucoma. Pilocarpine hydrochloride eyedrops are prescribed for her.

114. Mrs. Patterson asks the nurse what would have happened if she had ignored her symptoms. Which of the following statements would give Mrs. Patterson correct information?

    A. "You would lose your central vision."

    B. "Blindness can result if the condition is not treated."

    C. "The disease is progressive with or without treatment."

    D. "The lens would gradually become more opaque."

115. The pilocarpine eyedrops for Mrs. Patterson are expected to achieve which of these effects?

    A. To decrease drainage of aqueous humor from the posterior chamber of the eye.

    B. To control drainage of vitreous humor through the limbus of the eye.

    C. To promote drainage of aqueous humor through the canal of Schlemm.

    D. To prevent drainage of vitreous humor through the iris.

116. Mrs. Patterson should be impressed with the importance of taking the eyedrops as prescribed in order to prevent which of these complications?

    A. Distortion of the iris.

    B. Prolapse of the pupil.

    C. Spasm of the ciliary muscles.

    D. Damage to the optic nerve.

117. Mrs. Patterson should be instructed that pilocarpine eyedrops usually cause which of these temporary side effects?

A. Diplopia.

B. Blurring of vision.

C. Tinting of the sclera.

D. Color blindness.

---

Mrs. Mary Troy, 40 years old, is pregnant for the eighth time. She is attending the antepartal clinic. In her 16th week of gestation, she is to have an ultrasonogram and an amniocentesis.

---

118. Mrs. Troy is having the ultrasonogram before the amniocentesis for which of these purposes?

A. To locate the contents of the uterus.

B. To evaluate the muscle tone of the uterus.

C. To estimate the maturity of the fetus.

D. To test the reaction of the fetus to stress.

119. Mrs. Troy is having an amniocentesis performed in the 16th week of gestation for which of these purposes?

A. To evaluate the fetal environment.

B. To assess fetal age.

C. To determine the adequacy of antibody production in the fetus.

D. To identify abnormal chromosomal structure in the fetus.

---

At term, Mrs. Troy is admitted to the hospital in labor.

---

120. Mrs. Troy's contractions are 4 minutes apart, of 60 seconds' duration, and of moderate intensity. Her cervix is 5 cm. dilated. Mrs. Troy is in which of these phases of labor?

A. Preliminary.

B. Latent.

C. Active.

D. Transition.

---

Mrs. Troy delivers an 8-lb. (3,629-gm.) boy. Mrs. Troy is transferred to the postpartum unit and Baby Boy Troy is transferred to the nursery.

---

121. Because of her parity, Mrs. Troy is at greater risk to develop which of these problems in the fourth stage of labor?

A. A vaginal hematoma.

B. An elevated blood pressure.

C. Uterine atony.

D. Proteinuria.

122. On the first postpartum day after Mrs. Troy has seen and held her baby, she says to the nurse, "Could you feed him in the nursery? I'm so tired." The nurse should take which of these actions?

A. Carry out Mrs. Troy's request.

B. Encourage Mrs. Troy to feed the baby.

C. Record that Mrs. Troy is showing signs of poor maternal attachment.

D. Try to stimulate maternal bonding by feeding the baby in Mrs. Troy's room.

123. Mrs. Troy is considering the possibility of having a tubal ligation. A tubal ligation at this time will have which of these effects on the postpartum course?

A. The onset of regular menses will be delayed.

B. The production of ovarian hormones will decrease.

C. The involutional process will progress in its normal pattern.

D. The production of lochia rubra will be prolonged.

---

Roger Thomas, 15 years old, is seen in the mental health clinic for addiction to heroin. He is accompanied by his mother and his brother, Paul, who is 22 years old. The boys' father died 10 years ago.

---

124. During the initial interview, Paul says to the nurse, "I should have known something was wrong with Roger because he hasn't been himself lately. I could have helped him. We have been close since father died." The nurse's response should be determined by which of these interpretations of Paul's statement?

A. Paul is expressing guilt over his brother's drug problem.

B. Paul is concerned about the impact of his brother's drug use on his mother.

C. Paul is reporting that he failed as a role model for his brother.

D. Paul is blaming his brother's condition on the absence of a father.

125. To define the problem underlying Roger's dependence on heroin, the nurse should make which of these assessments initially?

A. The source of Roger's supply of heroin.

B. The conditions of Roger's social environment.

C. The level of Roger's academic achievement.

D. The effect of heroin on Roger's peer relationships.

126. Which of these comments, if made by Roger's mother, would demonstrate the best understanding of her son's situation?

A. "I guess I failed in teaching Roger the difference between right and wrong."

B. "I should not have protected Roger from situations that were discouraging for him."

C. "This would not have happened to Roger if I had remarried so he could have a father."

D. "My work schedule has kept me from giving Roger as much affection as he needs."

127. Roger behaves in a socially aggressive manner. It is most important to include which of these measures in his care?

A. Directing Roger to perform routine tasks.

B. Encouraging Roger to participate in team sport activities.

C. Maintaining set limits for Roger's behavior.

D. Restricting Roger's social interactions.

128. Roger begins to attend group psychotherapy sessions twice a week. The desired outcome of this therapy would be achieved when Roger starts to demonstrate which of these behaviors?

A. He identifies the effects of drugs on his personality.

B. He begins to deal with the effects of growing up without a father.

C. He develops insight into cause and effect in interpersonal relationships.

D. He resolves subconscious feelings of ambiguity about his mother.

Mrs. Grace Shaw, 44 years old, is admitted to the hospital with severe back pain. A herniated lumbar disc is suspected.

129. On admission, Mrs. Shaw states that she is having severe pain. Before an order for an analgesic is obtained, her care should include which of these measures?

A. Position her using trochanter rolls.

B. Raise the head of her bed to a high-Fowler's position.

C. Assist her to assume any position of comfort.

D. Elevate both of her feet on a pillow.

130. Mrs. Shaw is scheduled for a myelogram. Mrs. Shaw should be informed that a myelogram includes which of these procedures?

A. Electronic scanning.

B. Use of a contrast medium.

C. Injection of radioisotopes.

D. Ventricular monitoring.

Mrs. Shaw has a herniated disc, and a lumbar laminectomy is performed. She is brought to her room when her condition is stable.

131. To maintain the integrity of the surgical wound, Mrs. Shaw should be reminded to take which of these precautions?

A. "Do not rotate your ankles."

B. "Remember to flex and extend your hip every hour."

C. "Your torso must be moved as a unit."

D. "Try not to sneeze or cough."

132. In the early postoperative period, Mrs. Shaw must be given assistance with which of these measures?

A. Brushing her teeth.

B. Washing her face.

C. Washing her abdomen.

D. Cleansing her perineum.

133. On Mrs. Shaw's second postoperative day, she states, "I still have some of the same symptoms that I had before the surgery." The nurse should give Mrs. Shaw which of these explanations about her symptoms?

A. "The symptoms will persist, but you will require very little medication to conrol your pain."

B. "The symptoms will persist until the edema at the operative area subsides."

C. "The symptoms that are not relieved by surgery will be relieved by an injection of cortisone after the incision heals."

D. "The symptoms will persist until the nerve cells have time to regenerate."

This is the end of the test. Check to see whether you selected the correct answer to each question by using the answer key on page 204.

203

# Answer Key for Comprehensive Test Part I

| | | | | |
|---|---|---|---|---|
| 1. B | 28. D | 55. A | 82. A | 109. A |
| 2. D | 29. C | 56. D | 83. D | 110. D |
| 3. A | 30. B | 57. D | 84. D | 111. B |
| 4. C | 31. A | 58. C | 85. B | 112. A |
| 5. B | 32. A | 59. C | 86. A | 113. B |
| 6. C | 33. D | 60. B | 87. C | 114. B |
| 7. B | 34. C | 61. D | 88. D | 115. C |
| 8. C | 35. C | 62. C | 89. B | 116. D |
| 9. C | 36. A | 63. D | 90. B | 117. B |
| 10. B | 37. B | 64. B | 91. A | 118. A |
| 11. D | 38. B | 65. B | 92. C | 119. D |
| 12. D | 39. D | 66. Á | 93. B | 120. C |
| 13. A | 40. C | 67. C | 94. D | 121. C |
| 14. B | 41. C | 68. D | 95. C | 122. A |
| 15. A | 42. A | 69. A | 96. A | 123. C |
| 16. D | 43. B | 70. B | 97. C | 124. A |
| 17. B | 44. A | 71. C | 98. D | 125. B |
| 18. A | 45. B | 72. A | 99. D | 126. B |
| 19. A | 46. B | 73. A | 100. C | 127. C |
| 20. D | 47. C | 74. D | 101. D | 128. C |
| 21. D | 48. A | 75. B | 102. A | 129. C |
| 22. B | 49. D | 76. A | 103. C | 130. B |
| 23. A | 50. A | 77. A | 104. B | 131. C |
| 24. B | 51. C | 78. C | 105. A | 132. D |
| 25. C | 52. D | 79. A | 106. B | 133. B |
| 26. B | 53. C | 80. D | 107. C | |
| 27. D | 54. A | 81. B | 108. D | |

# COMPREHENSIVE TEST
## PART II

Read each question carefully. Select one answer from the four choices presented that you think answers the question correctly. There is only one correct answer to each question. Use the answer key on page 230 to find out whether the answer you selected is the correct one.

Mrs. Ida Asher, 76 years old, is admitted to the hospital with cancer of the lower sigmoid colon. She is scheduled for an abdomino-perineal resection. Her preoperative orders include a low-residue diet and neomycin sulfate orally.

----------------------------------------

1. The chief purpose of the low-residue diet preoperatively for Mrs. Asher is to

   A. prevent obstruction in the bowel.

   B. increase the peristaltic activity of the bowel.

   C. reduce the bulk of the bowel contents.

   D. promote healing of the bowel tissues.

2. Neomycin is administered to Mrs. Asher for which of these purposes?

   A. To minimize the formation of flatus in the intestines.

   B. To reduce the bacterial count in the intestines.

   C. To eliminate the need for repeated bowel irrigations.

   D. To prevent preoperative infection.

Mrs. Asher has the abdominoperineal resection. She has a colostomy appliance in place. When she is transferred to her room, she has an intravenous infusion running.

----------------------------------------

3. Mrs. Asher has serosanguineous drainage at the lower edge of her abdominal dressing. Before reporting this observation, it would be most important for the nurse to take which of these actions?

   A. Replace Mrs. Asher's dressing.

   B. Reinforce Mrs. Asher's dressing with a sterile dressing.

   C. Place an absorbent pad under Mrs. Asher.

   D. Reposition Mrs. Asher on her side so that the wound will drain by gravity.

4. The nurse notes that the area around the insertion site of Mrs. Asher's intravenous infusion is slightly edematous and that the intravenous fluids have stopped running. The nurse should make which of these interpretations of this finding?

   A. The vein into which the needle is inserted has collapsed.

   B. The apparatus has a defect.

   C. The fluid is being administered too rapidly.

   D. Fluids have infiltrated into the tissues.

206

5. Mrs. Asher is to sit in a chair for the first time. When helping Mrs. Asher to carry out the procedure, it would be essential for the nurse to take which of these actions?

   A. Select a chair for Mrs. Asher that has a firm seat.

   B. Reinforce Mrs. Asher's dressing before she gets out of bed.

   C. Have Mrs. Asher determine the time she prefers to get out of bed.

   D. Remain with Mrs. Asher to observe the effects of the procedure.

-----------------------------------------------------
Mr. Edward Dorman, 19 years old, is admitted to the hospital following a diving accident. He has an injury to the cervical spinal cord and a fracture at the level of C-6. His parents are notified. He is placed on a Stryker frame. Crutchfield tongs are applied. His orders include nothing by mouth, and an indwelling urethral catheter that is attached to gravity drainage.
-----------------------------------------------------

6. To turn Mr. Dorman while he is on the Stryker frame, it is essential for the nurse to include which of these actions in the procedure?

   A. Place straps around both frames before turning Mr. Dorman.

   B. Wrap Mr. Dorman's arms around the anterior frame during the turning.

   C. Remove the traction weights just before turning Mr. Dorman.

   D. Turn Mr. Dorman in a clockwise direction each time.

7. Mr. Dorman needs the urethral catheter because as an immediate outcome of his spinal cord injury, he will have which of these problems?

   A. Small bladder capacity.

   B. Hypertonic bladder.

   C. Frequent urinary tenesmus.

   D. Urinary retention.

8. When Mr. Dorman's parents arrive on the unit, the nurse explains their son's care to them. The nurse should give them which of these explanations about the purpose of the Crutchfield tongs?

   A. "They stimulate regeneration of cells in the spinal cord."

   B. "They help to keep the bones in the neck from pressing on nerves."

   C. "They assist in the prevention of swelling of the spinal cord."

   D. "They speed the healing of bones in the neck."

-----------------------------------------------------
The physician informs Mr. Dorman's parents that it is possible that Mr. Dorman will be permanently paralyzed from the neck down.
-----------------------------------------------------

9. After Mrs. Dorman is informed of her son's possible prognosis, she looks stunned. She paces up and down the corridor and repeatedly asks the nurse, "Will my son walk again?"

   After telling Mrs. Dorman that it is not known yet whether her son will walk, the nurse should take which of these approaches next?

   A. Ask Mrs. Dorman to explain what the physician told her.

   B. Have Mrs. Dorman sit down in a quiet place.

   C. Walk with Mrs. Dorman in the hallway.

   D. Tell Mrs. Dorman about her son's response to therapy thus far.

10. A diet as tolerated is ordered for Mr. Dorman. When giving him his first meal, the nurse should take which of these actions?

A. Give Mr. Dorman fluids before the solid foods.

B. Use a spoon to serve solid foods to Mr. Dorman.

C. Have an oropharyngeal suction machine at Mr. Dorman's bedside.

D. Place 2 pillows under Mr. Dorman's head.

11. Two weeks after his admission, Mr. Dorman adamantly refuses to be turned on the Stryker frame. The nurse should take which of these actions first?

A. Determine why Mr. Dorman is unwilling to be turned.

B. Tell Mr. Dorman that he should adhere to his turning schedule.

C. Explain to Mr. Dorman why he must be turned.

D. Ask Mr. Dorman how often he wants to be turned.

---------------------------------------------------
Four weeks after Mr. Dorman's injury, it is established that he had a total transection of the spinal cord at the C-6 level.
---------------------------------------------------

12. One day, when the nurse is washing Mr. Dorman's foot, his toes bend down. He says excitedly, "Did you see that? My toes moved! I'm beginning to be able to move now." The nurse's explanation to Mr. Dorman about the movement of his toes should include which of the following information?

A. The reflex activities are returning as a result of the lessening of spinal shock.

B. The parasympathetic nervous system is inhibiting skeletal muscle relaxation.

C. The sympathetic nervous system is initiating skeletal muscle contraction.

D. The initial paralysis is ending as a result of the decrease in edema of the spinal cord.

---------------------------------------------------
Mrs. Alma Bradley, 29 years old, is 4 months pregnant when she visits the antepartal clinic. The Bradleys have a son, Tom, who is 3 years old.
---------------------------------------------------

13. Mrs. Bradley says that she swims a half mile each day in an indoor pool. The nurse should give her which of the following information about swimming during her pregnancy?

A. Mrs. Bradley should continue to swim if Braxton Hicks contractions do not cause her discomfort.

B. Mrs. Bradley should swim a shorter distance.

C. Mrs. Bradley may continue to swim as long as she is comfortable doing so.

D. Mrs. Bradley must stop swimming during the last trimester of her pregnancy.

14. The nurse is discussing Mrs. Bradley's nutritional intake with her. Mrs. Bradley would demonstrate knowledge of foods containing protein and vitamin C if she selected which of these menus as <u>highest</u> in both nutrients?

A. Two barbecued frankfurters, potato salad, fresh grapes, chocolate milk.

B. A grilled hamburger on a bun, sliced tomato, coleslaw, a wedge of cantaloupe, whole milk.

C. Ham and cheese sandwich, cucumber salad, fresh sweet cherries, fresh lemonade.

D. Tuna fish and noodle casserole, dry toast, whipped gelatin dessert made with crushed pineapple, whole milk.

15. Mrs. Bradley and the nurse discuss pelvic
rocking exercises. An important purpose of
pelvic rocking exercises during pregnancy
is to

    A. distribute the fetus's weight equally
    within the abdominal cavity.

    B. decrease pressure on the bladder.

    C. relieve postural stress.

    D. increase uterine tone.

16. Which of these comments made by Mrs.
Bradley would best indicate that she is
achieving a psychological task of the
second trimester of pregnancy?

    A. "Becoming pregnant has made me feel more
    like a woman."

    B. "It wasn't a good time to become
    pregnant, but once I felt the baby move
    I really got excited."

    C. "With today's fashions, you can hardly
    tell that I'm wearing maternity clothes."

    D. "I've always been healthy, so I have no
    doubt that my baby will be healthy too."

At term, Mrs. Bradley is admitted to the
hospital. She is in early labor. Mrs. Bradley
develops dystocia. An intravenous infusion
containing oxytocin injection (Pitocin) is
started.

17. Pitocin should produce which of these
effects in Mrs. Bradley?

    A. An increase in the rate and force of
    uterine contractions.

    B. An increase in the force and a decrease
    in the frequency of uterine contractions.

    C. A decrease in uterine tone and in
    uterine sensitivity to thoracolumbar
    stimuli.

    D. A decrease in the duration and an
    increase in the frequency of uterine
    contractions.

18. Mrs. Bradley is observed for the effects of
Pitocin therapy. A marked alteration in
which of these vital signs would be most
indicative of an UNTOWARD effect of Pitocin
therapy?

    A. Pulse rate.

    B. Respirations.

    C. Temperature.

    D. Fetal heart tones.

19. Which of these symptoms in Mrs. Bradley
would be most indicative of Pitocin
overdosage?

    A. A contraction lasting more than
    2 minutes.

    B. Severe knifelike pain over the symphysis
    pubis.

    C. Dark red vaginal bleeding.

    D. Arrhythmic uterine contractions.

20. Meperidine (Demerol) hydrochloride 50 mg. and promethazine (Phenergan) hydrochloride 50 mg. are ordered for Mrs. Bradley. These drugs are expected to produce which of these effects in Mrs. Bradley?

A. Talkativeness and elevation of mood in spite of undiminished pain with contractions.

B. Relaxation and absence of pain with contractions.

C. Absence of pain and amnesia of events occurring before the administration of the medications.

D. Drowsiness but with awareness of contractions.

----------------------------------------

Mrs. Bradley's labor progresses, and she delivers a girl. Mrs. Bradley is transferred to the postpartum unit and Baby Girl Bradley is transferred to the nursery.

----------------------------------------

21. Mrs. Bradley tells the nurse that after her neighbor brought her baby home from the hospital, her preschooler demanded attention every time she began feeding the baby.

The nurse should suggest that if Mrs. Bradley's 3-year-old son demonstrates similar behavior, Mrs. Bradley should initially make which of these statements to him?

A. "We love you so much that we wanted to have another baby just like you."

B. "Soon you'll love the baby because you'll have someone to play with."

C. "I do have to take care of the baby a lot, but I love you and want to be with you too."

D. "You'll learn to love the baby if you help take care of her."

----------------------------------------

Jennifer Randall, 9 weeks old, is admitted to the hospital and has a surgical repair of a unilateral cleft lip. She has a cleft palate that will be repaired at a later date.

----------------------------------------

22. To meet Jennifer's emotional needs and to maintain the integrity of the surgical incision, which of these measures is essential in her early postoperative care?

A. Giving Jennifer a pacifier.

B. Responding to Jennifer as soon as she begins to cry.

C. Keeping elbow restraints on Jennifer.

D. Entertaining Jennifer with soft, colorful toys.

23. To feed Jennifer during the early post-operative period, it is important to use which of these utensils?

A. A soft nipple.

B. A plastic teaspoon.

C. A rubber-tipped medicine dropper.

D. A bulb syringe.

----------------------------------------

Jennifer is discharged, and when she is 18 months old she is admitted to the hospital for repair of the cleft palate.

----------------------------------------

24. During the admission interview with Jennifer's mother, Jennifer should be involved in which of these activities?

A. Jennifer should walk around the unit with a staff member.

B. Jennifer should be introduced to other children in the playroom.

C. Jennifer should remain with her mother.

D. Jennifer should be given toys to play with in her crib.

25. The report of Jennifer's blood tests includes the following results. Which one should be reported to the physician?

A. Hemoglobin, 9.4. gm. per 100 ml.

B. Leukocyte count, 7,200 per cu. mm. (mm$^3$).

C. Bleeding time, 60 seconds.

D. Erythrocyte count, 4,850,000 per cu. mm. (mm$^3$).

26. To plan play activities for Jennifer, the nurse should make which of these assessments of Jennifer?

A. Her developmental level.

B. Her response to toys shown to her.

C. Her familiarity with educational toys.

D. Her adjustment to hospitalization.

27. Since Jennifer most probably has fears common to children of her age, her care should include which of these measures?

A. Explaining equipment used in her care.

B. Repeating the purpose of her hospitalization.

C. Encouraging visits by her parents.

D. Allowing her the freedom to explore.

28. Jennifer has the repair of the cleft palate as scheduled. Her postoperative orders include acetaminophen (Tylenol) in liquid form. The medication should be administered by which of these methods?

A. Mixing the medication in applesauce and feeding it to Jennifer with a spoon.

B. Diluting the medication in 30 ml. of water and giving Jennifer a straw through which to sip it.

C. Measuring the medication in a medicine cup and having Jennifer drink it from the cup.

D. Mixing the medication with 60 ml. of orange juice and giving it to Jennifer in a bottle with a regular nipple.

---

Mr. Edward Rawley, 88 years old, has been living with his married son since becoming widowed five years ago. Mr. Rawley is brought to the clinic by his son because of increasing episodes of forgetfulness during which he accuses others of stealing from him.

---

29. During the initial interview with Mr. Rawley, it would be most important for the nurse to obtain the answer to which of the following questions?

A. What is the son's attitude toward his father?

B. What is the emotional climate in the son's home?

C. What is the pattern of dementia in Mr. Rawley's family?

D. What is Mr. Rawley's current physical status?

---

A psychiatric evaluation is arranged for Mr. Rawley, and a diagnosis of primary degenerative dementia is made. He is admitted to a skilled nursing facility.

---

30. During Mr. Rawley's adjustment to the skilled nursing facility, his care plan should emphasize which of these measures initially?

A. Reminding him to remain independent.

B. Adopting his usual daily routines to the fullest extent possible.

C. Encouraging his making friends through socialization.

D. Exploring his interest in diversional activities.

211

31. Mr. Rawley's son visits him several times during the first two weeks of Mr. Rawley's hospitalization. The son says to the nurse, "My father continues to refuse to talk with me. I had to let him be admitted. We couldn't keep him with us any longer."

To respond to the son's concerns at this time, which of these comments should the nurse make?

A. "It has been a difficult time for all of you."

B. "You have feelings of guilt about your father."

C. "You're having second thoughts about your decision."

D. "You did what you had to do under the circumstances."

32. A week later, when Mr. Rawley's son visits, Mr. Rawley tells him not to visit anymore. The son reports his father's statements to the nurse, and asks, "What should I do?" Which of these responses should the nurse make to best meet the needs of both the father and the son?

A. "You should wait a week or two to see if your father contacts you."

B. "You should continue to visit your father so that he knows you care about him."

C. "You might try phoning him every day instead of visiting with him here."

D. "Bring a friend with you the next time to make the visit easier for you."

33. Mr. Rawley is to be encouraged to increase his protein intake. Which of these nourishments would provide the highest amount of protein for him?

A. Cottage cheese and fruit.

B. Vanilla ice cream with strawberry sauce.

C. Chocolate milk.

D. Eggnog.

34. The nurse spends time with Mr. Rawley and recognizes that he confabulates. Mr. Rawley most probably uses confabulation for which of these purposes?

A. To express his sense of humor.

B. To protect his feelings of worth.

C. To control the topics of conversation.

D. To manipulate people.

35. The nurse is talking with Mr. Rawley and several other patients in the dayroom. Mr. Rawley suddenly gets up and heads for the door. He stops, and hangs his head. The nurse observes that Mr. Rawley has wet himself.

The nurse should take which of these actions?

A. Go to Mr. Rawley and say, "It's upsetting not to get to the bathroom in time. Let's get your clothes changed now."

B. Go to Mr. Rawley and say, "We'll get you on a schedule so this won't happen again. I'll get someone to help you change."

C. Say nothing and observe the manner in which Mr. Rawley deals with his crisis.

D. Avoid letting Mr. Rawley know that the nurse has observed his accident.

---------------------------------------------------
Mr. Robert Quinn, 52 years old, is admitted to the hospital with an acute myocardial infarction. He complains of chest pain, and his skin feels cold and clammy. His orders include a narcotic for relief of pain, and complete bed rest.
---------------------------------------------------

36. Mr. Quinn's chest pain is caused by which of these pathophysiological alterations that occur in myocardial infarction?

A. Congestion in the chambers within the heart.

B. Reduced oxygen supply to heart muscle.

C. Edema of affected heart tissue.

D. Retention of waste products in the heart.

37. When Mr. Quinn is admitted, the nurse should make which of these assessments first?

   A. Is Mr. Quinn having chest pain?

   B. What are Mr. Quinn's vital signs?

   C. Have blood studies been reported for Mr. Quinn?

   D. Does Mr. Quinn have a need for an infusion?

38. Mr. Quinn appears extremely apprehensive. After determining that he has received prescribed medication, the nurse should attempt to relieve his apprehension by taking which of these measures?

   A. Allowing Mr. Quinn to rest for a period without being disturbed.

   B. Explaining to Mr. Quinn the effects of stress on his present condition.

   C. Assuring Mr. Quinn that he will receive competent care.

   D. Giving Mr. Quinn information about the expected effect of his therapy.

39. Mr. Quinn has serum enzyme studies done daily. These studies are done for which of these purposes?

   A. To monitor the extent of myocardial damage.

   B. To evaluate biochemical activity in the myocardium.

   C. To monitor adequacy of blood flow to the myocardium.

   D. To determine the need for treatment to strengthen the myocardium.

40. If Mr. Quinn should develop ventricular tachycardia, the nurse should be prepared to administer which of these medications?

   A. Morphine sulfate.

   B. Digoxin (Lanoxin).

   C. Calcium gluconate.

   D. Lidocaine (Xylocaine) hydrochloride.

--------------------------------------------------
Mr. Quinn's condition is stable. He remains on bed rest. His orders include a low-sodium diet.
--------------------------------------------------

41. Mr. Quinn complains about the food he is being served. To meet Mr. Quinn's nutritional needs, the nurse should take which of these actions first?

   A. Determine Mr. Quinn's food likes and dislikes.

   B. Explain to Mr. Quinn the reason for the special diet.

   C. Suggest to Mr. Quinn that his family bring him food once a day.

   D. Inform Mr. Quinn that the diet prescription is a temporary therapeutic measure.

42. Although Mr. Quinn is ordered to be on bed rest, he gets out of bed and sits in a chair. To plan effective nursing intervention, the nurse should identify that Mr. Quinn is expressing which of these needs?

   A. He needs to be given explicit information about the possible effects of activity on his condition.

   B. He needs to have some control over his care to preserve his autonomy.

   C. He needs clear instruction to limit his regressed behavior.

   D. He needs the opportunity to deny that he is in a life-threatening situation.

213

---

Mrs. Laura Rigby, 38 years old, is transferred to the surgical unit following a right mastectomy. Several axillary nodes were excised. She has a wound catheter attached to a Hemovac.

---

43. Correct positioning of Mrs. Rigby's right arm is necessary to achieve which of these goals?

    A. To maintain strength in the abductor muscles.

    B. To minimize pressure on the incision.

    C. To promote lymphatic and venous drainage.

    D. To support the flexor and extensor muscles.

44. To promote the healing of Mrs. Rigby's surgical incision, the wound catheter is expected to have which of these effects?

    A. To increase capillary permeability in the incisional area.

    B. To drain transudate from the incisional area.

    C. To minimize pressure on the incisional area.

    D. To promte growth of granulation tissue in the incision.

45. To prevent a contracture in the right shoulder, Mrs. Rigby will be required to perform which of these exercises?

    A. Extension and flexion of the fingers and pronation of the forearm.

    B. Adduction and flexion of the elbow.

    C. Adduction and internal rotation of the shoulder.

    D. Abduction and external rotation of the shoulder.

46. Following Mrs. Rigby's discharge from the hospital, the optimal functioning of her right shoulder will be promoted if she performs which of these activities daily?

    A. Knitting.

    B. Carrying objects of increasing weight.

    C. Peeling potatoes.

    D. Drying dishes.

47. Mrs. Rigby should be instructed that she should perform breast self-examination at which of these times of her menstrual cycle?

    A. During ovulation.

    B. During the days immediately preceding menstruation.

    C. During menstruation.

    D. During the first few days after menstruation.

---

Mrs. Joan Unger, 22 years old, is accompanied by her husband when she is admitted to a psychiatric hospital. Mr. Unger reports being awakened at night by screams from his wife and finding her curled up in a corner, shouting that the house was being attacked by enemies. When he got close to his wife, she became combative. Mrs. Unger is assigned to a single room that is sparsely furnished. Plans are made for a nurse to remain with Mrs. Unger constantly.

---

48. Mrs. Unger's room assignment and nursing attention are planned to achieve which of these purposes?

    A. To simplify environmental stimuli and provide feedback to Mrs. Unger.

    B. To limit social contacts and allow Mrs. Unger to focus on her disability.

    C. To provide a role model for Mrs. Unger and teach her how to relate to others.

    D. To isolate Mrs. Unger and protect the other patients.

49. A one-to-one relationship is initiated with Mrs. Unger for which of these purposes?

   A. To redirect Mrs. Unger's aggressiveness into productive activities.

   B. To resolve Mrs. Unger's perceptions of injury by others.

   C. To identify Mrs. Unger's goals.

   D. To promote Mrs. Unger's independence.

50. Mrs. Unger is to receive a tranquilizer by mouth for extreme agitation; if refused, the medication is to be given intramuscularly. The nurse determines that Mrs. Unger needs the tranquilizer, but she refuses it. The nurse prepares the medication for intramuscular administration and arranges for two staff members to assist as necessary. The nurse should take which of these actions next?

   A. Have the assistants restrain Mrs. Unger while the injection is being given.

   B. Explain to Mrs. Unger the effects of the medication by injection.

   C. Ask Mrs. Unger to select the site to be used for the injection.

   D. Tell Mrs. Unger that the injection will be given to calm her.

51. Mrs. Unger is sitting with her back to the nurse. The nurse approaches and overhears her talking to an imaginary person. Mrs. Unger suddenly covers her ears and shouts, "I can't! I can't! "The nurse should take which of these actions?

   A. Call Mrs. Unger's name.

   B. Place a hand on Mrs. Unger's shoulder.

   C. Ask Mrs. Unger who she is speaking to.

   D. Continue to observe Mrs. Unger's behavior.

52. After several weeks, Mrs. Unger begins to trust the nurse who is assigned to her, and she complains about the relief staff person assigned to her when her primary nurse has days off. To support Mrs. Unger's right to her own opinion, which of these actions by the primary nurse would be supportive?

   A. Arrange a conference with Mrs. Unger and the staff person.

   B. Tell Mrs. Unger that another staff assignment will be made.

   C. Encourage Mrs. Unger to express her views.

   D. Explore with Mrs. Unger the reasons for her statements.

------------------------------------------------
Karla King, 8 months old, is admitted to the hospital with congestive heart failure that is related to a congenital cardiac defect. Karla is to be placed in a Croupette with oxygen. Her orders also include a low-sodium diet, a diuretic, and digoxin (Lanoxin).
------------------------------------------------

53. To determine the effectiveness of the diuretic for Karla, which of these measures should be taken?

   A. Recording her intake and output.

   B. Assessing the tenseness of her anterior fontanel.

   C. Weighing her every day.

   D. Testing her skin turgor.

54. Karla is to receive 0.045 mg. of Lanoxin twice a day. The bottle of Lanoxin contains 0.05 mg. per milliliter of solution. Karla should receive how many milliliters of the solution in each dose?

   A. 0.45

   B. 0.90

   C. 1.11

   D. 1.90

55. Which of these findings would be an early indication that Karla is responding to the digoxin therapy?

A. Her skin turgor is good.

B. Her cough is productive.

C. She sleeps 3 to 4 hours at a time.

D. Her urinary output has increased.


56. Four days after admission, the nurse takes Karla's apical pulse before administering the Lanoxin. Karla's apical pulse is 110 beats per minute. The nurse should take which of these actions?

A. Administer the medication and record the administration and the pulse rate.

B. Administer the medication, recheck the pulse rate in 30 minutes, and report the rate to the physician if it is below 110.

C. Withhold the medication and report the pulse rate to the physician.

D. Withhold the medication, recheck the pulse rate in 30 minutes, and administer the medication if the pulse rate is above 110.


57. Karla would have digoxin toxicity if she developed which of these symptoms?

A. Increased respiratory rate.

B. Refusal of feedings.

C. Dry mucous membranes.

D. Constipation.


58. Karla's developing sense of object permanence would be demonstrated by which of these behaviors?

A. Laughing aloud at her image in a mirror.

B. Putting her arms out to be picked up whenever a familiar person enters her room.

C. Uncovering a toy that she saw someone place under a blanket.

D. Biting anything that she can put into her mouth.


------------------------------------------------
Mrs. Evelyn Potter, 35 years old, has had gradually increasing menstrual bleeding and goes to see a physician. Mrs. Potter has two children, ages 4 and 6.
------------------------------------------------


59. Because Mrs. Potter has had excessive menstrual bleeding, the nurse should ask her which of these questions?

A. "Do you take tub baths during your period?"

B. "Have your periods usually been regular?"

C. "How many pads or tampons do you saturate each day during your period?"

D. "Have you changed from using tampons to using pads during your period?"


------------------------------------------------
Mrs. Evelyn Potter has multiple, large fibroids of the uterus and is admitted to the hospital for an abdominal hysterectomy.
------------------------------------------------


60. Before initiating Mrs. Potter's preoperative teaching, it would be most important for the nurse to make which of these assessments of Mrs. Potter?

A. Her level of anxiety.

B. Her ability to solve problems.

C. Her knowledge of the principles of learning.

D. Her previous experience with anesthesia.

61. Preoperatively, Mrs. Potter is taught deep-breathing and coughing exercises. The most reliable way of evaluating the effectiveness of the teaching would be to ask her which of these questions?

A. "Would you please describe the procedure for me, Mrs. Potter?"

B. "Will you please show me how you do the procedure, Mrs. Potter?

C. "What is the purpose of the procedure, Mrs. Potter?"

D. "Do you understand the procedure, Mrs. Potter?"

------------------------------------------------
Mrs. Potter has the surgery as planned. On the third day after surgery, Mrs. Potter develops a wound infection. A culture and sensitivity testing of the wound is done. She is to be started on cephalothin sodium (Keflin) therapy.
------------------------------------------------

62. The sensitivity testing of Mrs. Potter's wound is done for which of these purposes?

A. To identify the susceptibility of the causative microorganism to the action of antibiotics.

B. To determine the virulence of the microorganism causing the infection.

C. To identify antibiotics to which Mrs. Potter is allergic.

D. To determine if Mrs. Potter has any antibodies against the microorganism causing the infection.

63. During the time that Mrs. Potter's wound has drainage, it would be most important that her care include which of these measures?

A. Wearing a mask when entering her room.

B. Using an aerosol disinfectant spray in her room.

C. Sealing her soiled dressings in a waterproof bag.

D. Securing a waterproof cover over her freshly applied sterile dressing.

64. Before giving Mrs. Potter her first dose of Keflin, it would be most important for the nurse to take which of these actions?

A. Inquire if she ever took a sulfa drug.

B. Advise her not to consume milk products while receiving this medication.

C. Tell her not to be alarmed if her urine turns reddish-orange because of this medication.

D. Ask her if she ever had a reaction to penicillin.

------------------------------------------------
Mrs. Potter's wound infection responds to treatment. She is being prepared for discharge. Ferrous sulfate is ordered for her.
------------------------------------------------

65. The nurse should instruct Mrs. Potter that the absorption of iron will be improved if the ferrous sulfate is taken with

A. an antacid.

B. orange juice.

C. milk.

D. water.

66. An iron-rich diet is ordered for Mrs. Potter. In discussing the diet with Mrs. Potter, the nurse should instruct her that the iron content is highest in which of these foods?

A. Cheese.

B. Yogurt.

C. Raisins.

D. Strawberries.

---
Mrs. Connie Dunne, a 24-year-old primigravida, has received antepartal care from a private physician. At term, she is admitted to the labor and delivery unit of the hospital. She is having contractions every 5 minutes.
---

67. Which of these behaviors by Mrs. Dunne would be most characteristic of nearing the end of the first stage of labor?

    A. She says, "I'm so hungry."

    B. She screams, "I can't take this anymore!"

    C. She moans quietly during contractions.

    D. She listens attentively to the nurse's instructions.

68. Mrs. Dunne will have reached the end of the first stage of labor when which of these observations is made?

    A. The cervix is completely dilated.

    B. The membranes have ruptured.

    C. Uterine contractions are occurring every 1 to 2 minutes.

    D. The infant is delivered.

---
Mrs. Dunne delivers an apparently normal boy weighing 7 lb. 4 oz. (3,289-gm.) over an episiotomy. Baby Boy Dunne is to be bottle-fed and to room-in with Mrs. Dunne. They are both transferred to the postpartum unit.
---

69. Mrs. Dunne is very elated and talkative when she is returned to the postpartum unit. In view of Mrs. Dunne's emotional state, which of these actions should be taken?

    A. Acknowledge Mrs. Dunne's feelings and continue to listen to her.

    B. Prepare Mrs. Dunne for sleep and leave the room.

    C. Remind Mrs. Dunne to conserve her energy.

    D. Give Mrs. Dunne a sedative.

70. On Mrs. Dunne's first postpartum day, she says to the nurse, "My stitches hurt." Which of these actions should the nurse take first?

    A. Give Mrs. Dunne perineal care.

    B. Examine Mrs. Dunne's perineum.

    C. Instruct Mrs. Dunne to relax the perineal area.

    D. Ask Mrs. Dunne if she wants an analgesic.

71. Baby Boy Dunne's birth weight was 7 lb. 4 oz. (3,289-gm.). When he is 3 days old, he weighs 7 lb. (3,175-gm.). Mrs. Dunne says, "I'm worried about my baby's weight loss." The nurse should make which of these responses?

    A. "Most babies lose weight during their first few days because of fluid shifts."

    B. "Babies lose weight because they are not yet able to metabolize their formula."

    C. "We'll ask the doctor to increase the strength of the baby's formula."

    D. "Perhaps the baby should be fed at more frequent intervals."

72. Mrs. Dunne says to the nurse, "How long will my baby have the soft spot at the front of his head?" The nurse's reply should inform Mrs. Dunne that the anterior fontanel usually is closed by how many months after birth?

    A. 3

    B. 8

    C. 13

    D. 18

Mr. Sam Tucker, 63 years old, is admitted to the hospital with moderately advanced emphysema. His orders include oxygen by nasal cannula at 2 liters per minute, and postural drainage.

73. Mr. Tucker has arterial blood gas analysis. Respiratory acidosis in Mr. Tucker would be confirmed by which of these test results?

A. Decreased carbon dioxide, increased pH, and increased bicarbonate levels.

B. Increased carbon dioxide, decreased pH, and increased bicarbonate levels.

C. Decreased carbon dioxide, decreased pH, and decreased bicarbonate levels.

D. Increased carbon dioxide, increased pH, and decreased bicarbonate levels.

74. Mr. Tucker should be observed for symptoms of respiratory acidosis, which include

A. diaphoresis.

B. elevated temperature.

C. drowsiness.

D. deep respirations.

75. Mr. Tucker's order for oxygen limits the amount to 2 liters per minute to prevent which of these effects on him of a higher concentration of oxygen?

A. Depressing his stimulus for breathing.

B. Stimulating his production of pulmonary surfactant.

C. Increasing his pulmonary pressure.

D. Collapsing his alveolar membranes.

76. Oxygen therapy for Mr. Tucker is expected to have which of these effects?

A. To decrease the viscosity of his sputum.

B. To increase the productivity of his cough.

C. To stimulate diaphragmatic breathing.

D. To reduce his respiratory effort.

77. During postural drainage, to drain secretions from the posterior basal segment of Mr. Tucker's right lung, he should be placed in which of these positions?

A. On his back, with the head of the bed elevated.

B. On his back, with the foot of the bed elevated.

C. On his left side, with the head of the bed elevated.

D. On his left side, with the foot of the bed elevated.

78. After Mr. Tucker has completed postural drainage, it is most important to include which of these measures in his care?

A. Giving him mouth care.

B. Offering him a warm drink.

C. Having him perform deep-breathing exercises.

D. Monitoring his pulse rate.

Mrs. Delores Owens, 28 years old, is seen in the clinic because of symptoms of hyper-thyroidism. She is scheduled for diagnostic tests.

79. While preparing to take a nursing history from Mrs. Owens, the nurse should expect to make which of these observations of Mrs. Owens?

A. She will have a fine tremor of her hands.

B. She will have dry, scaly skin.

C. She will be sitting quietly without talking to other patients.

D. She will be overweight.

80. If Mrs. Owens has hyperthyroidism, she will have which of these symptoms?

A. Brittle hair.

B. Lethargy.

C. Palpitations.

D. Poor appetite.

81. Mrs. Owens is to have all of the following diagnostic tests. Which one will require that she return for a scan over the thyroid to determine results?

A. Triiodothyronine ($T_3$).

B. Levothyroxine ($T_4$).

C. Protein-bound iodine (PBI).

D. Radioactive iodine uptake (RAI).

Results of diagnostic tests for Mrs. Owens conclude that she has a growth in the thyroid that is causing the hyperthyroidism. She is to be treated with methimazole (Tapazole) before being scheduled for surgery.

82. Tapazole is prescribed for Mrs. Owens to achieve which of these expected effects?

A. To reduce the size of the thyroid gland.

B. To achieve an euthyroid state.

C. To lower levels of the thyroid-stimulating hormone.

D. To encapsulate the tumor.

Three months later, Mrs. Owens is admitted to the hospital for a subtotal thyroidectomy. Her orders include saturated solution of potassium iodide (SSKI).

83. Mrs. Owens is to receive SSKI for which of these purposes?

A. To increase her serum potassium level.

B. To promote excretion of iodide.

C. To reduce the vascularity of the thyroid gland.

D. To control the production of the thyroid hormone.

84. Preoperatively, Mrs. Owens should be taught how she should support her neck following surgery to prevent stress on the incision. Which of these demonstrations would be correct?

A. Raise the elbows and place both hands behind the neck.

B. Place both hands on the side of the face and apply slight pressure.

C. Put one hand on the chin and the other hand against the back of the head.

D. Pull both shoulders backward and hyperextend the head.

Mrs. Owens has a subtotal thyroidectomy. She is brought to the recovery room, and when her condition is stable, she is transferred to her room.

85. After Mrs. Owens is transferred to her bed, she should be placed in which of these positions?

A. Right side-lying, with one pillow under her head and shoulders.

B. Semi-Fowler's, with the head supported by pillows.

C. Supine, with the head on the bed without pillows.

D. Sitting erect, with pillows on an overbed table on which to lay her head.

86. To assess Mrs. Owens for effects of edema surrounding the recurrent laryngeal nerve, the nurse should take which of these actions?

A. Have Mrs. Owens try to cough.

B. Instruct Mrs. Owens to yawn.

C. Ask Mrs. Owens to speak.

D. Observe Mrs. Owens's ability to swallow.

87. An early development of hypoparathyroidism in Mrs. Owens would be indicated by which of these symptoms?

A. Twitching of the hands.

B. Flank pain.

C. Elevated serum calcium levels.

D. Pallor.

Angela Saum, 8 years old, is admitted to the hospital with acute rheumatic fever. Her orders include bed rest, and aspirin four times a day.

88. Since Angela has acute rheumatic fever, she most probably has which of these symptoms?

A. Migratory joint pain.

B. Hematuria.

C. Pedal edema.

D. Anemia.

89. Angela's acute rheumatic fever was most probably diagnosed on the basis of the result of which of these tests?

A. Complete blood count.

B. Antistreptolysin O titer.

C. Electrocardiogram.

D. Urine culture.

90. Since Angela is to receive aspirin several times a day, it is most important to add which of these measures to her care plan?

A. Offering fluids containing vitamin C.

B. Increasing intake of foods high in vitamin K.

C. Monitoring pedal pulses.

D. Checking for evidence of petechiae.

91. To plan appropriate activities for Angela while she is on bed rest, the nurse should consider which of these characteristics of school-age children?

A. They require a sense of achievement.

B. They have a limited attention span.

C. They are developing muscular coordination.

D. They display volatile personalities.

92. To monitor Angela for possible side effects of aspirin, her care plan should include which of these measures?

A. Testing her hearing.

B. Calculating her daily urine output.

C. Monitoring her blood pressure.

D. Evaluating her pedal pulses.

---

Angela's condition improves, and plans are made for her discharge. She is to receive prophylactic penicillin therapy at home.

---

93. When discussing plans for Angela's discharge with the nurse, Mrs. Saum asks about measures required to prevent Angela from infecting the two other children in the family. The nurse should include which of the following information about precautions to be taken at home?

A. Disposable dishes and utensils should be used to serve meals to Angela.

B. Careful handwashing should be carried out after direct contact with Angela.

C. Angela should be isolated from other members of the family as much as possible.

D. No restrictions will be required in Angela's contacts with members of the family.

94. Angela is to receive penicillin prophylactically for which of these purposes?

A. To hasten the elimination of toxins related to infectious processes.

B. To develop an antigen-antibody response to respiratory infections.

C. To alter the body's autoimmune reaction to viral infections.

D. To prevent a recurrence of streptococcal infections.

---

Mr. Fred Oakley, 38 years old and married, is brought to the hospital. He is disheveled and smells strongly of alcohol. His clothing is torn and he has several abrasions on his head and face. He was found by the police, who saw him staggering about in a park. Since he has head injuries, he is admitted to the hospital for observation. Mr. Oakley's wife has been notified and she arrives to see him.

---

95. After Mrs. Oakley visits briefly with her husband, she says to the nurse, "I've told him that his drinking binges would get him in trouble. He won't listen and I've done everything I can to help him. No one can blame me." The nurse should interpret Mrs. Oakley's statements as communicating which of these messages?

A. She came to see her husband because she was called by the authorities.

B. She is severing her relationship with her husband.

C. She feels helpless in dealing with her husband's behavior.

D. She is embarrassed by her husband's drunkenness.

96. When discussing Mr. Oakley's drinking problem with his wife, the nurse should attempt to convey that persons who experience episodes of excessive drinking usually have which of these behavioral problems?

A. Boredom.

B. Insecurity.

C. Confusion.

D. Insensitivity.

Mr. Oakley is admitted to a center for the treatment of alcohol abuse. He admits to having drunk at least a liter of alcohol every day for the past several weeks.

Mr. Oakley's symptoms of alcohol withdrawal decrease. He is resistant to participating in group therapy and states that he can manage without help at this time.

97. In anticipation of Mr. Oakley's developing withdrawal symptoms, the nurse should consider which of these environmental factors?

   A. The proximity of resuscitation equipment.

   B. The adequacy of lighting.

   C. The availability of belts, shoelaces, and the like.

   D. The distance to the bathroom.

98. The next morning Mr. Oakley is alert and oriented. He says to the nurse, "I don't remember what happened yesterday, but I guess I behaved pretty badly." Which of these responses by the nurse would best protect Mr. Oakley's self-esteem?

   A. "You were not responsible for your actions."

   B. "You should not think about yesterday's events."

   C. "You're wondering how you behaved yesterday."

   D. "Staff members do not take offense at hearing abusive language."

99. Mr. Oakley begins to hallucinate and he is tremulous. At this time, which of these measures would be most important for Mr. Oakley?

   A. Remaining with him.

   B. Explaining the temporary nature of his symptoms.

   C. Assessing his orientation to reality.

   D. Encouraging him to drink fruit juices.

100. Although Mr. Oakley resists the efforts of staff members to talk with him, the staff continues to attempt to find ways of communicating with him. The efforts of the staff are planned to achieve which of these goals?

   A. To closely monitor Mr. Oakley's activities.

   B. To convince Mr. Oakley of the dangers of alcoholism.

   C. To demonstrate belief in Mr. Oakley's worth as a person.

   D. To obtain information about Mr. Oakley's plans to avoid alcohol.

101. Which of these comments, if made by Mr. Oakley, would most strongly indicate that he understands his problem?

   A. "I must limit my drinking to a measured amount once a week."

   B. "I will stay away from all my friends who could convince me to have one more drink."

   C. "Having just one drink will lead me into my old drinking habits."

   D. "I will never drink except for a glass of wine with dinner."

102. Mr. Oakley is improved. To best facilitate his rehabilitation after his discharge, which of these measures would be most important?

A. Determining his wife's commitment to helping him.

B. Planning nonalcohol-related recreational activities for him.

C. Arranging for him to participate in a community program devoted to helping others.

D. Evaluating the psychosocial environment to which he will return.

---

Mr. Walter Young, 60 years old, has a history of hoarseness. He is admitted to the hospital for a direct laryngoscopy and biopsy.

---

103. Mr. Young is anxious about the possible results of the laryngoscopy and he makes references to having cancer. To be supportive of Mr. Young, which of these statements by the nurse would be most therapeutic?

A. "Try not to worry about the test, because it is a routine examination."

B. "I understand your concern as the results can be frightening."

C. "You seem worried about the outcome of the examination."

D. "Perhaps you would like to call your doctor to talk more about your condition."

104. Mr. Young has the laryngoscopy. After he is brought to his room, he says he is thirsty. Before giving him fluids, the nurse should determine the answer to which of these questions?

A. What is Mr. Young's diet order?

B. Can Mr. Young extend his tongue?

C. Has Mr. Young's gag reflex returned?

D. What does Mr. Young want to drink?

---

Mr. Young is scheduled for a laryngectomy and a neck dissection. The surgical procedure has been explained to Mr. Young and his wife.

---

105. Mrs. Young is with her husband when the nurse enters his room. Mrs. Young says, "My husband thinks he may not be accepted by his friends when he returns to work because he will be disfigured." The nurse should take which of these actions?

A. Describe for the Youngs how clothing can be worn to cover the stoma.

B. Encourage the Youngs to talk about their concerns.

C. Inform the Youngs that they will have a conference about rehabilitative measures before Mr. Young is discharged from the hospital.

D. Explain how participation in meetings of patients with Mr. Young's problem will help him make necessary adjustments in his life.

---

Mr. Young has surgery as scheduled. When his condition is stable, he is brought back to his unit. He has a laryngectomy tube in place. His orders include nasogastric tube feedings.

---

106. In the immediate postoperative period, Mr. Young's care plan should give priority to which of these measures?

A. Restoring electrolyte balance.

B. Maintaining patency of the airway.

C. Promoting comfort through position changes.

D. Dealing with altered body image.

107. Mr. Young is to have nasogastric tube feedings rather than oral feedings primarily for which of these purposes?

A. To prevent aspiration.

B. To decrease salivation.

C. To prohibit swallowing.

D. To promote healing.

---

Kenneth Potter, 12 years old, is admitted to the hospital in sickle cell crisis. His knees and ankles are swollen and painful. Kenneth was 2 years old when the diagnosis of sickle cell anemia was made. His orders include an analgesic for relief of pain.

---

108. In addition to giving Kenneth prescribed medication for relief of pain, the nurse should most certainly carry out which of these measures?

A. Performing passive range-of-motion exercises of Kenneth's legs.

B. Assisting Kenneth to assume a position of comfort.

C. Monitoring Kenneth's vital signs.

D. Encouraging Kenneth to eat foods high in vitamin C.

109. If Kenneth has reduced renal concentrating ability, he will have which of these symptoms?

A. Nocturia.

B. Hematuria.

C. Dysuria.

D. Pyuria.

110. While Kenneth is acutely ill, which of these measures will promote resolution of the vaso-occlusive crisis?

A. Massaging the involved joints.

B. Applying cold compresses to the affected areas.

C. Encouraging a high fluid intake.

D. Performing active exercises of the extremities.

111. The acute onset of Kenneth's sickle cell crisis was caused by which of these physiological alterations?

A. Accumulation of abnormal blood cells in small blood vessels.

B. Overproduction of erythrocytes in bone marrow.

C. Destruction of blood cells in the spleen.

D. Decreasing ability of hemoglobin to carry oxygen.

112. When Kenneth is feeling better, he says to the nurse, "My older brother has the sickle cell trait. Why doesn't he have crises like I do?" The nurse's response should include which of the following information about persons who have the sickle cell trait?

A. They require a diet of foods high in iron to prevent symptoms.

B. They develop symptoms if they exercise strenuously.

C. They may have acute episodes in adulthood.

D. They usually exhibit no symptoms of the disease.

Mrs. Margaret Evans, 64 years old, has extensive peripheral vascular disease due to arteriosclerosis. She is admitted to the hospital with gangrene of the left toes.

113. When performing a physical assessment of Mrs. Evans's left leg, the nurse should expect that which of these pulses will be diminished most?

A. Femoral.

B. Popliteal.

C. Posterior tibial.

D. Dorsalis pedis.

Mrs. Evans has a midthigh amputation of her left leg. Her condition is stable when she is brought back to her room.

114. In the immediate postoperative period, Mrs. Evans should be observed for the complication that is most common following an amputation of a lower extremity, which is

A. fat embolism.

B. hemorrhage.

C. sloughing of sutures.

D. tissue necrosis.

115. If appropriate measures are not taken, Mrs. Evans will be prone to which of these complications of the affected extremity?

A. Internal rotation of the stump.

B. Abduction of the stump.

C. Flexion contracture of the left hip.

D. Muscle spasms of the left thigh.

116. When Mrs. Evans's suture line on the stump has healed sufficiently, stump care is taught to her. Which of these observations of her stump will indicate that the desired results of stump care are achieved?

A. The stump has an apparent keloid forming.

B. The stump has a callous.

C. The skin on the stump is tough and pliable.

D. The skin on the stump feels soft and lubricated.

117. Mrs. Evans begins to walk with crutches. When Mrs. Evans is walking with the crutches, immediate correction would be required if the nurse were to make which of these observations?

A. Mrs. Evans's elbows are slightly flexed when she is holding the hand bars.

B. Mrs. Evans advances both crutches before taking a step with her right foot.

C. Mrs. Evans holds the crutches snugly under her axillae.

D. Mrs. Evans glances down at the floor before proceeding to take a step.

118. Mrs. Evans's left leg is fitted with a prosthesis. She is to avoid bearing weight on the affected extremity. Mrs. Evans should be taught to use which of these methods of walking with crutches?

A. Advancing the affected extremity and both crutches while bearing weight on the unaffected leg.

B. Advancing the unaffected leg and left crutch while bearing weight on the right leg and right crutch.

C. Advancing the right leg and left crutch while bearing weight on the right crutch.

D. Advancing the unaffected leg while bearing weight on both crutches.

119. One day Mrs. Evans says to the nurse, "It would be easier to be dead than go through all this. I'll never be able to go back to work or do things that I had planned." The nurse's response should be based on which of these interpretations of Mrs. Evans's statement?

A. She is experiencing depression as a result of the loss of a valued part of her body.

B. She is in a state of disbelief regarding her amputation.

C. She is using rationalization to deal with her altered body image.

D. She is beginning to accept the full extent of her disability.

---------------------------------------------

Mr. Edward Waller, 40 years old, is a computer programmer. He believes that his behavior is being controlled by buttons pushed by his employer and that his thoughts are being recorded. After he refused to go to work for a week, his wife contacted the family physician, who helped to arrange Mr. Waller's admission to a psychiatric hospital.

---------------------------------------------

120. Soon after admission, a nurse enters Mr. Waller's room and sits down near him. Mr. Waller jumps up, dashes out of the room, and says angrily, "Why am I here? I'm not staying. Keep away from me." The nurse should make which of these interpretations of Mr. Waller's behavior?

A. He has never been in a hospital before.

B. He is fearful of the nurse's intentions.

C. He is hallucinating.

D. He believes that he is unlikely to benefit from treatment.

121. On admission, which of these goals should be the chief basis of planning care for Mr. Waller?

A. To foster his self-evaluation.

B. To promote his resocialization.

C. To provide him with intense environmental stimulation.

D. To strengthen his self-control.

122. To begin to establish a trusting relationship with Mr. Waller, the nurse should use which of these approaches?

A. Encouraging Mr. Waller to talk about anything he wishes.

B. Focusing Mr. Waller on objective reality when his remarks become irrational.

C. Telling Mr. Waller the purpose served by suspicion of others.

D. Discussing ways Mr. Waller could begin to understand the behavior of others.

123. A few days after Mr. Waller was admitted, a newly employed nurse asks Mr. Waller about his background and interests. Mr. Waller replies angrily, "Why are you trying to get all this information from me? Isn't it on my record?" To respond to Mr. Waller, the nurse should make which of these statements?

A. "I'm sorry you don't feel like talking, Mr. Waller."

B. "I can look at your chart if you prefer, Mr. Waller."

C. "There's no reason to distrust me, Mr. Waller."

D. "You value your privacy, don't you, Mr. Waller."

124. One day Mr. Waller is in the dayroom talking with the nurse when a young female patient stops at the doorway wearing only her nightgown. Mr. Waller says to the nurse angrily, "She's half naked! Do something or else I will!" The nurse should make which of these interpretations of Mr. Waller's outburst?

A. He is asking the nurse if the patient's attire is acceptable.

B. He dislikes the female patient.

C. He wants the nurse to agree with his opinion of the patient.

D. He is asking the nurse to help him deal with his unconscious impulses.

---
Mrs. Emma Ganz, 55 years old, has a history of cirrhosis. She is admitted to the hospital following an episode of hematemesis.
---

125. Mrs. Ganz has blood studies done. The results indicate that she has a prolonged prothrombin time. Because of this, Mrs. Ganz should be observed for the possible development of which of these symptoms?

A. Pruritis.

B. Paresthesia.

C. Jaundice.

D. Ecchymosis.

---
Mrs. Ganz vomits a large amount of bright red blood. An esophageal tamponade (Blakemore tube) is inserted and attached to low, intermittent suction.
---

126. While Mrs. Ganz has the Blakemore tube in place, her care will require which of these measures?

A. Suctioning oropharyngeal secretions when necessary.

B. Assessing bowel sounds every 2 hours.

C. Testing the gastric drainage for the presence of blood every 4 hours.

D. Deflating the esophageal balloons for 5 minutes every 24 hours.

127. Mrs. Ganz begins to have periods of confusion, and she refuses to follow simple directions. The nasogastric tube is draining coffee-ground material. The nurse should make which of these interpretations of Mrs. Ganz's behavior?

A. The action of intestinal bacteria on digested blood is causing her level of serum ammonia to increase.

B. The volume of her blood loss is causing symptoms of hypovolemic shock.

C. The extent of her liver disease is beginning to interfere with the clotting of her blood.

D. The decrease in her circulating body fluid has disturbed her electrolyte balance.

128. Mrs. Ganz is to be observed for symptoms of impending hepatic coma. The development of hepatic coma would be indicted by which of these symptoms?

A. Fetid odor of her breath.

B. Flapping hand tremors.

C. Kussmaul's breathing.

D. Restlessness.

129. Mrs. Ganz's serum bilirubin increases, and she has signs of jaundice. To control pruritus, which of these measures should be added to her care plan?

A. Applying antiseptic lotion to the skin.

B. Dusting the skin with talcum powder.

C. Sponging the skin with tepid water.

D. Massaging the skin with mineral oil.

------------------------------------------------
The remainder of the questions are individual questions.
------------------------------------------------

130. A pregnant woman has an incompetent cervical os. She has a surgical procedure performed to suture the cervix closed. Because she has had this procedure, she should be instructed to take which of these actions?

A. Avoid taking tub baths.

B. Refrain from sexual intercourse.

C. Irrigate her vagina with a normal saline solution.

D. Notify the physician if she has any signs of labor.

131. A woman who is carrying twins is in labor. Her contractions are 3 minutes apart. One of the fetal heart rates is 98 immediately after a contraction and returns to 120 one minute before the onset of the next contraction.

After positioning the woman on her side, which of these actions should the nurse take first?

A. Notify the physician.

B. Compare this fetal heart rate with the heart rate of the second fetus.

C. Advise the woman to take shallow breaths.

D. Check the woman's blood pressure.

132. In a neonate, symptoms of withdrawal from an addictive drug such as heroin include

A. hyperglycemia.

B. hyperbilirubinemia.

C. hyperthermia.

D. hypertonicity.

This is the end of the test. Check to see whether you selected the correct answer to each question by using the answer key on page 230.

# Answer Key for Comprehensive Test Part II

| | | | | |
|---|---|---|---|---|
| 1. C | 28. C | 55. D | 82. B | 109. D |
| 2. B | 29. D | 56. A | 83. C | 110. C |
| 3. B | 30. B | 57. B | 84. A | 111. A |
| 4. D | 31. A | 58. C | 85. B | 112. D |
| 5. D | 32. B | 59. C | 86. C | 113. D |
| 6. A | 33. D | 60. A | 87. A | 114. B |
| 7. D | 34. B | 61. B | 88. A | 115. C |
| 8. B | 35. A | 62. A | 89. B | 116. C |
| 9. C | 36. B | 63. C | 90. D | 117. C |
| 10. C | 37. A | 64. D | 91. A | 118. A |
| 11. A | 38. D | 65. B | 92. A | 119. A |
| 12. A | 39. A | 66. C | 93. D | 120. B |
| 13. C | 40. D | 67. B | 94. D | 121. D |
| 14. B | 41. A | 68. A | 95. C | 122. B |
| 15. C | 42. B | 69. A | 96. B | 123. D |
| 16. B | 43. C | 70. B | 97. B | 124. D |
| 17. A | 44. B | 71. A | 98. C | 125. D |
| 18. D | 45. D | 72. D | 99. A | 126. A |
| 19. A | 46. D | 73. B | 100. C | 127. A |
| 20. D | 47. D | 74. C | 101. C | 128. B |
| 21. C | 48. A | 75. A | 102. D | 129. C |
| 22. B | 49. B | 76. D | 103. C | 130. D |
| 23. C | 50. D | 77. D | 104. C | 131. A |
| 24. C | 51. A | 78. A | 105. B | 132. D |
| 25. A | 52. C | 79. A | 106. B | |
| 26. A | 53. C | 80. C | 107. D | |
| 27. C | 54. B | 81. D | 108. B | |

# Registry

Commission on Graduates of Foreign Nursing
 Schools
3624 Market Street
Philadelphia, Pennsylvania   19104

National Council of State
 Boards of Nursing, Inc.
625 North Michigan Avenue - Suite 1544
Chicago, Illinois   60611

National League for Nursing
10 Columbus Circle
New York, New York   10019

## BOARDS OF NURSING

ALABAMA
Executive Officer
Alabama Board of Nursing
Suite 203, 500 Eastern Boulevard
Montgomery, Alabama   36117

ALASKA
Executive Secretary
Alaska Board of Nursing
Department of Commerce and Economic Development
Division of Occupational Licensing
The Frontier Building
3601 C Street, Suite 722
Anchorage, Alaska   99502-0333

AMERICAN SAMOA
Executive Secretary
American Samoa Health Service
 Regulatory Board
Pago Pago, American Samoa   96799

ARIZONA
Executive Director
Arizona State Board of Nursing
5050 N. 19th Avenue, Suite 103
Phoenix, Arizona   85015

ARKANSAS
Executive Director
Arkansas State Board of Nursing
Westmark Building, Suite 308
4120 W. Markham Street
Little Rock, Arkansas   72205

CALIFORNIA
Executive Officer
California Board of Registered Nursing
1030 - 13th Street, Suite 200
Sacramento, California   95814

COLORADO
Program Administrator
Colorado Board of Nursing
State Services Building, Room 132
1525 Sherman Street
Denver, Colorado   80203

CONNECTICUT
Executive Officer
Connecticut Board of Examiners for Nursing
150 Washington Street
Hartford, Connecticut   06106

DELAWARE
Executive Director
Delaware Board of Nursing
Margaret O'Neill Building
P.O. Box 1401
Dover, Delaware   19901

DISTRICT OF COLUMBIA
President
District of Columbia Board of Nursing
614 H Street, N.W.
Washington, DC   20001

FLORIDA
Executive Director
Florida Board of Nursing
111 Coastline Drive, East
Jacksonville, Florida   32202

GEORGIA
Executive Director
Georgia Board of Nursing
166 Pryor Street, S.W.
Atlanta, Georgia   30303

GUAM
Nurse Examiner Administrator
Guam Board of Nurse Examiners
Department of Public Health and Social Services
P.O. Box 2816
Agana, Guam   96910

HAWAII
Executive Secretary
Hawaii Board of Nursing
P.O. Box 3469
Honolulu, Hawaii  96801

IDAHO
Executive Director
Idaho Board of Nursing
Hall of Mirrors
700 West State Street
Boise, Idaho  83720

ILLINOIS
Nursing Education Coordinator
Department of Registration and Education
320 West Washington Street
3rd Floor
Springfield, Illinois  62786

INDIANA
Board Administrator
Indiana State Board of Nurses' Registration
  and Nursing Education
Health Professions Service Bureau
964 North Pennsylvania Street
Indianapolis, Indiana  46204

IOWA
Executive Director
Iowa Board of Nursing
Executive Hills East
1223 East Court
Des Moines, Iowa  50319

KANSAS
Executive Administrator
Kansas Board of Nursing
503 Kansas Avenue, Suite 330
P.O. Box 1098
Topeka, Kansas  66601

KENTUCKY
Executive Director
Kentucky State Board of Nursing
4010 Dupont Circle, Suite 430
Louisville, Kentucky  40207

LOUISIANA
Executive Director
Louisiana State Board of Nursing
150 Baronne Street, Room 907
New Orleans, Louisiana  70112

MAINE
Executive Director
Maine State Board of Nursing
295 Water Street
Augusta, Maine  04330

MARYLAND
Executive Director
Maryland Board of Examiners of Nurses
201 West Preston Street
Baltimore, Maryland  21201

MASSACHUSETTS
Executive Secretary
Board of Registration in Nursing
Leverett Saltonstall Building
100 Cambridge Street
Boston, Massachusetts  02202

MICHIGAN
Nursing Consultant
Michigan Board of Nursing
Department of Licensing and Regulation
Ottawa Towers North
611 West Ottawa
P.O. Box 30018
Lansing, Michigan  48909

MINNESOTA
Executive Secretary
Minnesota Board of Nursing
717 Delaware Street, S.E.
Minneapolis, Minnesota  55414

MISSISSIPPI
Executive Director
Mississippi Board of Nursing
135 Bounds Street, Suite 101
Jackson, Mississippi  39206

MISSOURI
Executive Director
Missouri State Board of Nursing
P.O. Box 656
3523 N. Ten Mile Drive
Jefferson City, Missouri  65102

MONTANA
Executive Secretary
Montana State Board of Nursing
Department of Commerce
Division of Business and Professional Licensing
1424 9th Avenue
Helena, Montana  59620-0407

NEBRASKA
Associate Director
Board of Nursing
Bureau of Examining Boards
Department of Health
State House Station
P.O. Box 95007
Lincoln, Nebraska  68509

NEVADA
Executive Director
Nevada State Board of Nursing
1281 Terminal Way, Suite 116
Reno, Nevada  89502

NEW HAMPSHIRE
Executive Director
New Hampshire Board of Nursing Education
  and Nurse Registration
State Department of Education
State Office Park South
101 Pleasant Street
Concord, New Hampshire  03301

NEW JERSEY
Executive Director
New Jersey Board of Nursing
1100 Raymond Boulevard, Room 319
Newark, New Jersey  07102

NEW MEXICO
Executive Director
New Mexico Board of Nursing
4125 Carlisle N.E.
Albuquerque, New Mexico  87108

NEW YORK
Executive Secretary
New York State Board for Nursing
State Education Department
Cultural Education Center, Room 3013
Albany, New York  12230

NORTH CAROLINA
Executive Director
North Carolina Board of Nursing
P.O. Box 2129
Raleigh, North Carolina  27602

NORTH DAKOTA
Executive Director
North Dakota Board for Nursing
Kirkwood Office Tower, Suite 504
7th Street South
Bismarck, North Dakota  58501

NORTHERN MARIANA ISLANDS
Chairperson
Commonwealth Board of Nurse Examiners
P.O. Box 1458
Saipan, CM  96950

OHIO
Executive Secretary
Ohio Board of Nursing Education
  and Nursing Registration
65 South Front Street
Suite 509
Columbus, Ohio  43215

OKLAHOMA
Executive Director
Oklahoma Board of Nurse Registration
  and Nursing Education
2915 N. Classen Boulevard
Suite 524
Oklahoma City, Oklahoma  73106

OREGON
Executive Director
Oregon State Board of Nursing
1400 S.W. 5th Avenue, Room 904
Portland, Oregon  97201

PENNSYLVANIA
Executive Secretary
Pennsylvania State Board of Nurse Examiners
Department of State
P.O. Box 2649
Harrisburg, Pennsylvania  17105

RHODE ISLAND
Executive Secretary
Rhode Island Board of Nurse Registration
  and Nursing Education
Health Department Building
75 Davis Street, Room 104
Providence, Rhode Island  02908

SOUTH CAROLINA
Executive Director
State Board of Nursing for South Carolina
1777 St. Julian Place, Suite 102
Columbia, South Carolina  29204

SOUTH DAKOTA
Executive Secretary
South Dakota Board of Nursing
304 S. Phillips Avenue, Suite 205
Sioux Falls, South Dakota  57102

TENNESSEE
Executive Director
Tennessee State Board of Nursing
283 Plus Park Boulevard
Nashville, Tennessee  37216

TEXAS
Executive Secretary
Board of Nurse Examiners for the State of Texas
1300 Anderson Lane, Building C
Suite 225
Austin, Texas  78752

UTAH
Executive Secretary and Nurse Consultant
Utah State Board of Nursing
Division of Registration
Heber M. Wells Building, 4th Floor
160 East 300 South
P.O. Box 5802
Salt Lake City, Utah  84110

VERMONT
Executive Director
Vermont State Board of Nursing
Redstone Building
26 Terrace Street
Montpelier, Vermont  05602

VIRGIN ISLANDS
Chairperson
Virgin Islands Board of Nurse Licensure
Division of Professional Licensing
P.O. Box 7309
Charlotte Amalie
St. Thomas, Virgin Islands  00801

VIRGINIA
Executive Secretary
Virginia State Board of Nursing
P.O. Box 27708
Richmond, Virginia  23261

WASHINGTON
Executive Secretary
Washington State Board of Nursing
Division of Professional Licensing
P.O. Box 9649
Olympia, Washington  98504

WEST VIRGINIA
Executive Secretary
West Virginia Board of Examiners for
 Registered Nurses
922 Quarrier Street
Suite 309, Embleton Building
Charleston, West Virginia  25301

WISCONSIN
Director
Wisconsin Bureau of Nursing
Department of Regulation and Licensing
P.O. Box 8936
Madison, Wisconsin  53708

WYOMING
Executive Director
Wyoming State Board of Nursing
2223 Warren Avenue
Suite 1 - 2nd Floor
Cheyenne, Wyoming  82002

## Your Opinion, Please?

This study guide was developed to assist you in preparing to take NCLEX-RN and other tests used in nursing. We are interested in knowing whether the information provided was helpful to you. Won't you please take a few minutes to let us know your opinion? Please make your comments as specific as possible. We will be very pleased to hear from you.

COMMENTS:_____

_____

_____

_____

_____

_____

_____

_____

_____

_____

_____

_____

Please mail to: Leonarda A. Laskevich
               National League for Nursing
               10 Columbus Circle
               New York, New York 10019